A Practical Guide to Respiratory System and its Related Disorders

Kemal M. Surji

978-1-62265-932-6 (online)

978-1-62265-933-3 (paper)

About the Author

Kemal Surji is a professor of healthcare administration in public and private institutions. For more than 20 years he has practiced respiratory therapy and taught courses in medical, health and management related fields at both the undergraduate and graduate levels. He is the author of several publications in diversified academic fields. Additionally, Dr. Surji has worked as a consultant and advisor in a variety of related areas. Including healthcare program development, educational programs enhancement, medical practice improvement and patient satisfaction perfection and improve quality and care.

Dr. Surji received his undergraduate degree in 1990, Board Certification, and Registry to practice Respiratory medicine/therapy in 1993 from the state of Tennessee USA; Board Certification of Pulmonary Technology and Prenatal/Pediatric Specialty in 1994. Masters of Science degree in Community Health/ Wellness Promotion in 2003, PhD in Health Administration in 2005 and Public Health in 2008 with over 20 years of academic and educational experience in different academics and health settings.

Preface

This textbook is intended to offer the healthcare students and providers such as medical students, respiratory and nursing practitioners as well as allied health professionals with fundamentals of respiratory system, assessments and diagnostic procedures in pulmonary medicine. Furthermore, the subsequent chapters of the text, present the most common disorders of respiratory system, each chapter is designed to specify a specific respiratory disorder in a comprehensive format as follows:

- Description of each disorder
- The pathologic changes of the lungs
- The main symptoms for individual conditions
- The etiologic factors of disorders
- Chest assessment and diagnostic procedures
- Treatment and medications
- End of chapter review questions

This textbook provides subject material on clinical respiratory problems in an effective manner made to order for busy physicians and other health care providers. The discussions for individual topics are short, and selected chapters are accompanied by a commentary that presents supplemental information or an experienced view.

The content of the book is based upon the authors years of practice as a respiratory practitioner and hospital based clinical educator in the filled of pulmonary care. As an educator, the author has taken under consideration the magnitude of student needs and learning style. Students are not attracted to busy homework assignments and long lectures regarding information they can obtain through internet. The students also become very impatience with boring textbooks having no user-friendly and comprehensible applications. They become more involved and retain information that are embedded in experiential learning and connected to personal experience.

The degree to which the content of the text is relevant, practical, and applicable to the real situation is a critical issue. Students of healthcare are willing to invest time and effort into textbooks that help them accomplish their goal. Information that are applicable and concise presented in a practical application framework are well acknowledged by the students.

Students in the medical field of respiratory education desire to understand what is the disorder, what are the symptoms, what causes the condition and how to diagnose and treat it. This textbook is designed to aid student through critical thinking, experiential learning method that links the classroom to the real world.

Acknowledgements

Preparation of this textbook would not have been possible without the students' criticism of the boring and difficult to understand course books in general. Therefore, a special appreciation goes to all the healthcare and medical students in the region. Special thanks to all the doctors, nurses and allied health practitioners for their hard work and dedication in saving lives every day.

Kemal Surji PhD, RRT

Contents

Preface ii

Chapter 1 1

    Basic Understanding of Respiratory System 2

    Reason to Breathe 3

    Aerobic Respiration 4

    Upper respiratory tract: 5

    Lower respiratory tract: 5

    Physiology of Breathing 10

    The Respiratory Pathways 15

    Oxygen transport 16

    Blood Oxygen Content 17

    The Bohr Effect 18

    The Haldane effect 19

    Review Questions 20

Chapter 2 21

    Respiratory Assessment 22

    Assessment of the Chest 23

    Chest Inspection 23

    Patterns of Breathing 26

    Ventilation-Perfusion Ratio (V/Q) 35

    Ventilatory Disturbances 36

    Ventilation Regulation 37

    Chemoreceptors 37

    Receptors of the Lung 40

    Dedicated Respiratory Centers In The Lower Brain Stem 42

    Pulmonary Shunt 43

    Anatomic shunt 44

    Capillary shunt 44

    Shunt-like effect or Relative shunt 45

    Shunt Equation 47

    Lung compliance 49

    Airway Resistance 51

    A Cough and Sputum Production 52

Hemoptysis 55

Barrel Chest or Increased Anteroposterior Chest Diameter 57

Pursed-Lip Breathing (PLB) 58

Polycythemia, Cor-Pulmonale 61

Digital Clubbing 64

Arterial Blood Gasses 65

Acid-Base Balance- pH 72

Pulmonary Function Test (PFT) 81

Electrocardiogram (EKG) Monitoring 93

Electrophysiology of the Heart 94

Arrhythmias 96

Review Questions 101

Common Respiratory Disorders 102

Chapter 3 103

Chronic Cough 104

Mechanism of Cough 104

Etiologic Factors of a Chronic Cough 105

Treatment of Chronic Cough 106

Review Questions 110

Chapter 4 111

Asthma 113

Pathologic Changes of the Lungs 113

Most Common Visible Symptoms of Asthma 114

Cardiac symptoms of asthma: 115

Etiologic Factors of Asthma 115

The Immunologic Mechanism 116

Chest Assessments and Diagnostic Findings 119

Treatment of Asthma 121

Patient Education 126

MDI Teaching Method 126

Review Questions 128

Chapter 5 129

Chronic Bronchitis 131

Pathologic Changes of the Lungs 131

The Major Symptoms of Chronic Bronchitis..132

Etiologic Factors of Chronic Bronchitis 132

Chest Assessments and Diagnostic Findings 133

Treatment of Chronic Bronchitis 135

Review Questions 140

Chapter 6 141

Emphysema 142

Pathologic Changes of the Lung with Emphysema 142

The Major Symptoms of Emphysema 143

Etiologic Factors of Emphysema Disease...143

Chest Assessment and Diagnostic Findings 144

Treatment of Emphysema...147

Review Questions 152

Chapter 7 153

Chronic Obstructive Pulmonary Disease COPD 155

Pathologic Changes of the Lung with COPD 155

The major Symptoms of COPD..156

Etiologic Factors of COPD...156

Chest Assessment and Diagnostic Findings 157

Treatment of COPD..160

Surgery to Treat COPD 166

Review Questions 167

Chapter 8 168

Bronchiectasis..170

Pathologic Changes of the Lung with Bronchiectasis 170

The major Symptoms of Bronchiectasis 171

Etiologic Factors of Bronchiectasis 172

Chest Assessment and Diagnostic Findings 173

Treatment of Bronchiectasis 177

Review Questions 183

Chapter 9 183

Pneumonia 185

Pathologic Changes of the Lung with Pneumonia 186

The major Symptoms of Pneumonia 186

Etiologic Factors of Pneumonia 187

Chest Assessment and Diagnostic Findings of Pneumonia 190

Treatment of Pneumonia 193

Review Questions 196

Chapter 10 197

Pulmonary Edema 198

Pathologic Changes of the Lung with Pulmonary Edema 198

The major Symptoms of Pulmonary Edema 198

Etiologic Factors of Pulmonary Edema 199

Chest Assessment and Diagnostic Findings of Pulmonary Edema 201

Treatment of Pulmonary Edema 203

Review Questions 207

Chapter 11 208

Acute (Adult) Respiratory Distress Syndrome 210

Pathologic Changes of the Lung with ARDS 210

The Major Symptoms of ARDS 211

Etiologic Factors of ARDS 211

Chest Assessment and Diagnostic Findings of ARDS 212

Treatment of ARDS 214

Review Questions 216

Chapter 12 217

Flail Chest 219

Pathologic Changes of the Lung with Flail Chest 219

The major Symptoms of Flail Chest 220

Etiologic Factors of Flail Chest 220

Chest Assessment and Diagnostic Findings of Flail Chest 221

Treatment of Flail Chest 222

Review Questions 223

Chapter 13 224

Pneumothorax 226

Pathologic Changes of the Lung with pneumothorax 226

The main symptoms of pneumothorax 227

Etiologic Factors of pneumothorax 227

Chest Assessment and Diagnostic Findings 229

Treatment of pneumothorax 231

Review Questions 232

Chapter 14 233

Pleural Effusion 235

Pathologic Changes of the Lung with Pleural effusion.. 235

The major Symptoms of Pleural Effusion 235

Etiologic Factors of Pleural Effusion... 236

Chest Assessment and Diagnostic Findings of Pleural Effusion 238

Treatment of Pleural Effusion... 241

Review Questions 243

Chapter 15 244

Pulmonary Embolism (PE) 246

Pathologic Changes of the Lung with Pulmonary Embolism 246

The major Symptoms of Pulmonary Embolism 247

Etiologic Factors of Pulmonary Embolism.. 247

Chest Assessment and Diagnostic Findings of Pulmonary Embolism 248

Treatment of Pulmonary Embolism.. 253

Review Questions 255

Chapter 16 256

Tuberculosis... 258

Pathologic Changes of the Lung with Tuberculosis 259

The Major Sign and Symptoms of Tuberculosis 259

Etiologic Factors of Tuberculosis... 261

Chest Assessment and Diagnostic Findings 262

Treatment of Tuberculosis... 266

Review Questions 268

Chapter 17 269

Croup Syndrome 271

Pathologic Changes of the Lung with Croup Syndrome....................................... 271

The major Symptoms of Croup Syndrome 272

Etiologic Factors of Croup Syndrome and Epiglottitis 273

Chest Assessment and Diagnostic Findings 274

Treatment of Croup Syndrome 276

Review Questions 279

Chapter 18 280

    Cystic Fibrosis 282

    Pathologic Changes of the Lung with Cystic Fibrosis 282

    The major Symptoms of Cystic Fibrosis 284

    Etiologic Factors of Cystic Fibrosis 285

    Chest Assessment and Diagnostic Findings 287

    Treatment of Cystic Fibrosis 289

    Review Questions 295

Chapter 19 296

    Sleep Apnea 298

    The stages of sleep apnea: 298

    The Three Types of Sleep Apnea 300

    The Major Symptoms of Sleep Apnea 302

    Methods of Evaluation of Sleep Apnea 304

    Diagnostics Procedures to Evaluate the Sleep Apnea 306

    Treatment of Sleep Apnea 309

    Review Questions 313

Chapter 20 314

    Cancer of The Lung 316

    Pathologic Changes of the Lung with Carcinoma 316

    The main symptoms of Lung Cancer 316

    Etiologic Factors of Lung Cancer 318

    Types of Lung Cancer 319

    Chest Assessment and Diagnostic Findings 319

    Treatment of Lung Cancer 324

    Review Questions 327

References 328

Glossary of Most Common Respiratory Terminology 352

Appendixes 356

    Appendix I Abbreviations 356

    Appendix II Respiratory Therapy Equations 357

Index 359

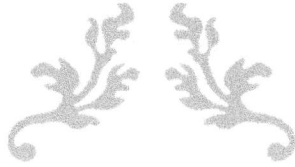

Chapter 1

Basic Understanding of Respiratory System

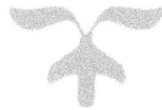

Chapter Objectives

1. Explain the reason to breathe
2. Describe aerobic respiration
3. Illustrate and define respiratory anatomy and physiology

Nasal Cavity

Pharynx

Larynx

Trachea

Bronchioles

Lungs

Bronchi

Alveoli

Diaphragm

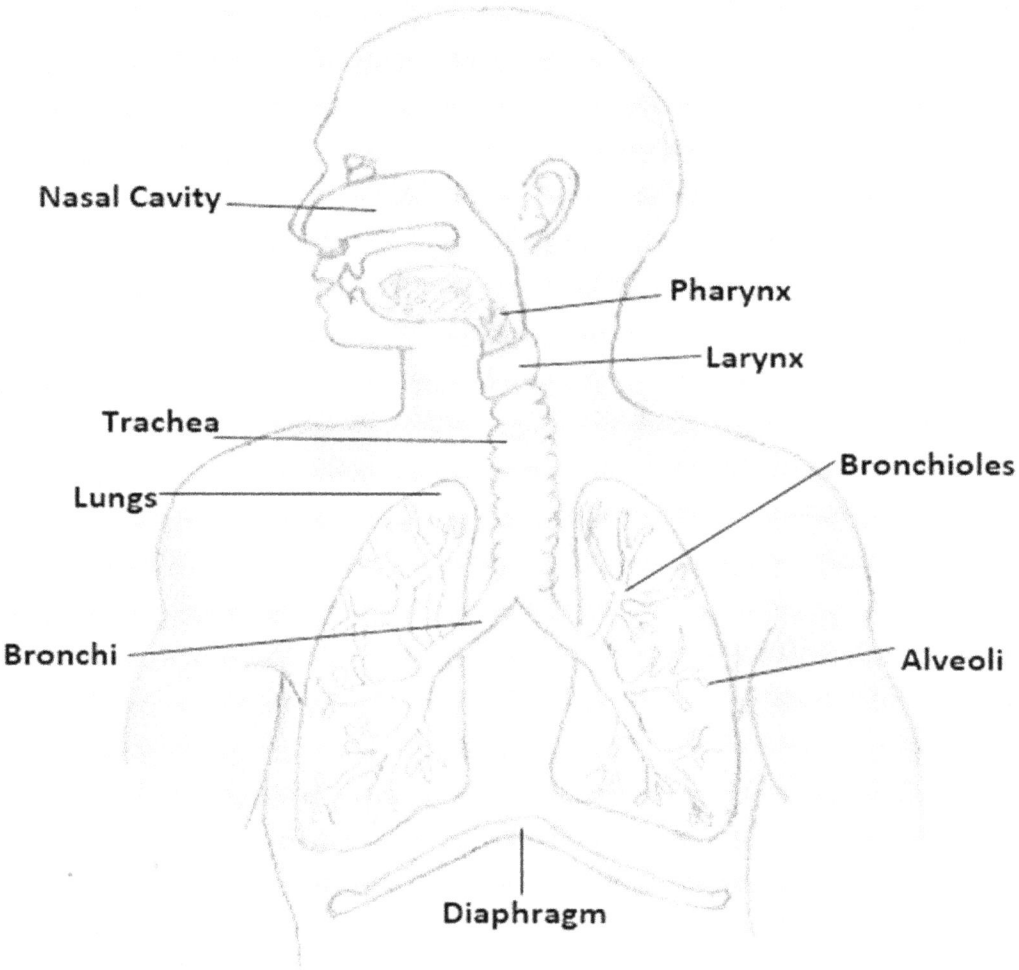

Figure 1-1 Illustrates the anatomy of respiratory system

Reason to Breathe

The reason for breathing is to live. Therefore, to live, a constant supply of energy needed in the cells.

The following process is required to produce energy:

➢ consuming food with carbohydrates
➢ Ability to convert carbohydrates to glucose (sugar)
➢ Ability to convert glucose to energy. (Glucose must combine with oxygen to release the energy to the cells).
➢ Ability to inhale oxygen while breathing.

The aerobic respiration equation for the above process is as follows:

Glucose + Oxygen → Energy + Carbon Dioxide + Water

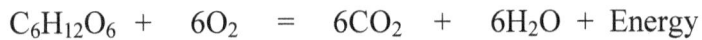

$$C_6H_{12}O_6 + 6O_2 = 6CO_2 + 6H_2O + Energy$$

The process of aerobic respiration, as shown above, takes place in a section of a cell called mitochondria. Figure 1-2 illustrates the aerobic respiration:

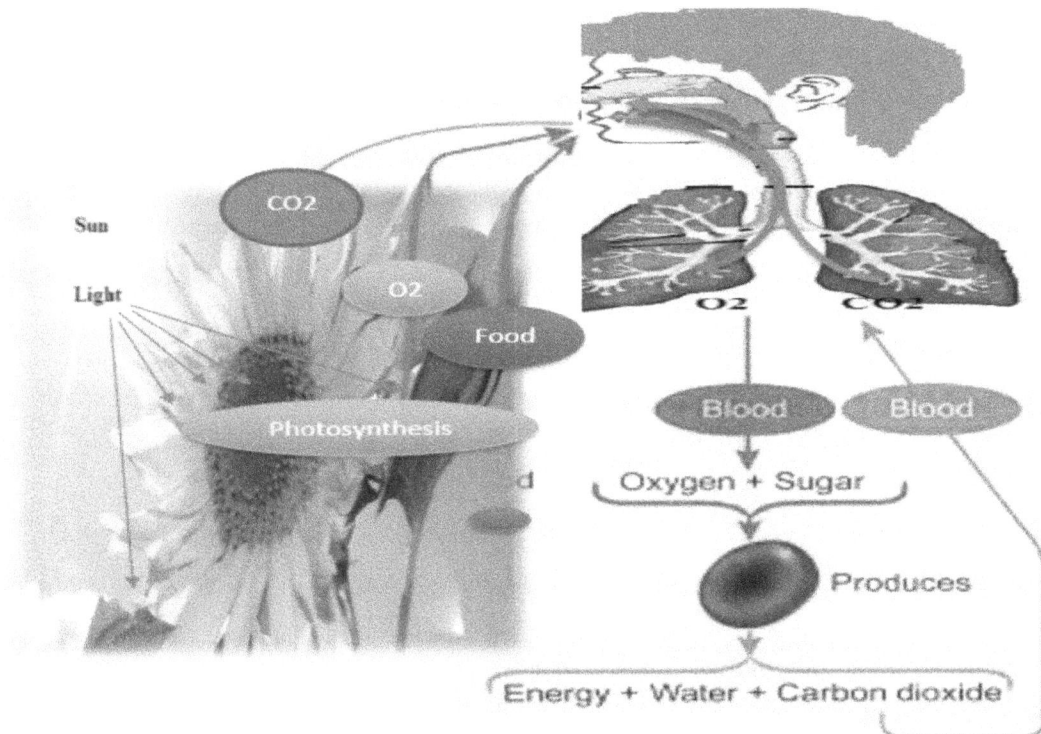

Figure 1-2 shows the aerobic respiration

The process of the aerobic respiration equation indicates that glucose uses oxygen to burn and release energy. Thereby, producing two waste products as carbon dioxide and water known as metabolic wastes. Carbon dioxide and water as wastes will diffuse out of the cells and enter the blood then move into the alveoli of the lungs for exhalation. These wastes of carbon dioxide and water are exhaled as carbon dioxide gas and water vapor during expiration.

Therefore, the two significant reasons to breathe are:

➢ To inhale oxygen to burn food for energy.
➢ To breathe out carbon dioxide gas and water vapor that are waste products as food is converted into energy. Without energy, the body cells cannot live.

Respiratory Anatomy and Physiology

The entire tissues within the body require oxygen to function. The purpose of the respiratory system, which comprises air passageways, the lungs, pulmonary vessels, and respiratory muscles, delivers oxygenated blood to the body tissues and removes waste gasses. Therefore, The respiratory system assists the body in the exchange of gasses between the outside air, blood, and the body's billions of cells. Distribution of air aided by the most of the organs of the respiratory system. However, only the tiny, grape-like alveoli and the alveolar ducts handle the actual gas exchange.

Along with air distribution and gas exchange, the respiratory system filters, warms, and humidifies the air to breathe. Certain organs in the respiratory system also play a part in the sense of smell and speech. The respiratory system assists the body to sustain homeostasis or balance amongst the various elements of the internal environment of the body.

Summary of the fundamental function of the respiratory system:

- Filters, warms and humidifies outside air before inhalation
- Exchange of gasses between outside air and the lungs
- Diffusion of oxygen via the alveoli and alveolar ducts into the blood
- Distribution of oxygen binding to hemoglobin into the tissues
- Dissemination of the wasted product as carbon dioxide to the lungs for removal
- Assist in the sense of smell and speech
- Help in maintaining homeostasis

The two primary elements of the respiratory system are upper respiratory tract and lower respiratory tract:

Upper respiratory tract:

The organs are positioned outside the chest cavity and Comprised of the nose, the pharynx, and the larynx.

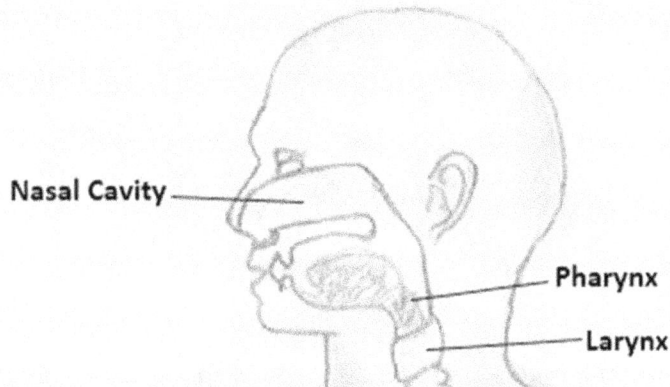

Figure 1-3 displays the upper respiratory tract consists of a nasal cavity, pharynx, and larynx.

- **The nasal cavity** is the upper respiratory tract's first organ. Within the nose, the sticky lubricated mucous membrane coating the nasal cavity that traps dust particles. Additionally, there are tiny hairs called cilia aid to move dust particles to the nose to be sneezed or blown out. Therefore, Nasal Cavity is a system of cavities with a mucous membrane that air passes through from the nostrils to the pharynx as the breathing air is strained, warmed, moistened, and sensed. The pharynx is a hollow tube approximately 10 cm long that begins from behind the nose and ends at the upper trachea (windpipe). If one were to breathe through the mouth, air would enter the pharynx.
- **Sinuses**: These air-filled spaces alongside the nose aid in making the skull lighter.
- **The pharynx** is a passageway for both food and air before getting to their suitable destinations. Moreover, the pharynx plays a role in speech as well.
- **Larynx**: The larynx is vital to human speech and it is called voice box.

Lower respiratory tract:

All the organs of the lower respiratory tract found inside the chest cavity. Lower respiratory tract includes the trachea, the lungs, and all segments of the bronchial tree including the alveoli.

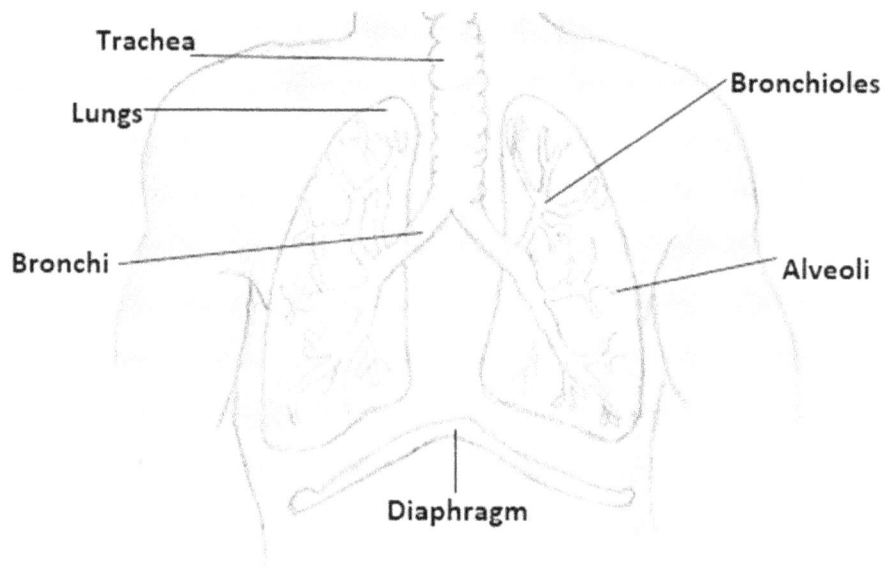

Figure 1-4 Displays the lower respiratory system including trachea, right and left lungs, bronchi, bronchioles, alveoli, and diaphragm.

- **Trachea**: Found just below the larynx, the trachea is the main airway to the lungs. Another name for trachea is the windpipe. The trachea is a wide pipe that is kept open by C-shaped rings of tough tissue. It is the passageway through which air passes. The trachea has a mucous membrane for trapping dust and germs and moving them towards pharynx.

- **Epiglottis** is a flexible flap at the root of the tongue that shields the tracheal opening while swallowing so that food does not enter the trachea (windpipe).

- **Lungs**: Together the lungs shapes one of the body's largest organs. Lungs are responsible for providing oxygen to capillaries to be distributed to the tissues and exhaling carbon dioxide. The makeup of the lungs includes the bronchial tree, air tubes branching off from the bronchi into the smaller segmental bronchus and further smaller air tubes known as bronchiole, each one ending in a pulmonary alveolus.

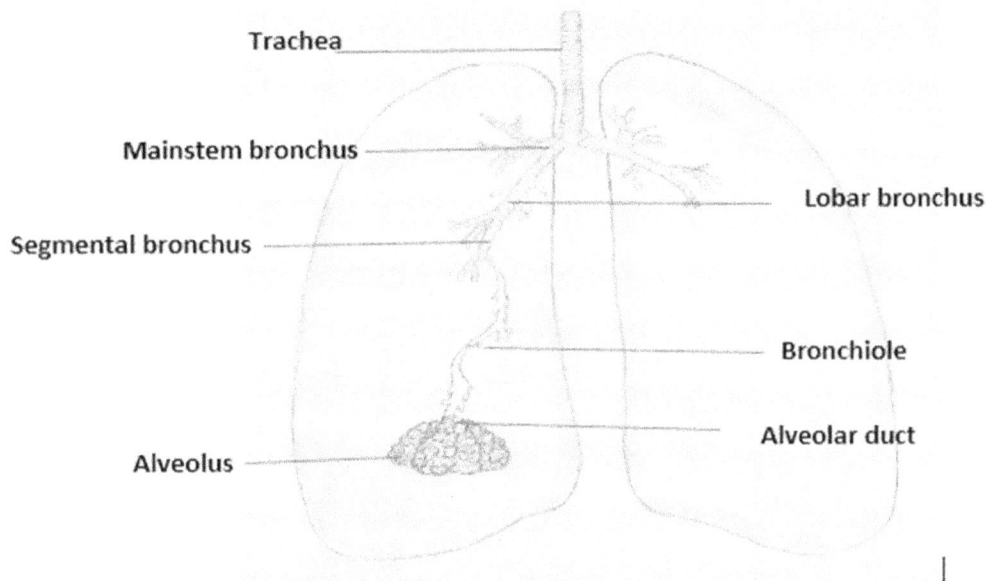

Figure 1-5 Illustration of tracheobronchial tree

- **Bronchi:** As the trachea approaches the lungs, at the carina, it subdivides into two branches. The left and right bronchus. Plural of the bronchus is bronchi. Each bronchus joins to a separate lung. The bronchi lined with mucous membranes for trapping dust and microscopic particles such as germs. The bronchi are also kept open by C-shaped rings of tough tissue.

- **The Bronchiole** as the bronchi extend further into the lungs they subdivide into many smaller tubes called bronchioles that end in the pulmonary alveolus. The bronchioles found in the lungs. Bronchioles do not have the C-shaped rings of tough tissue, but they are just tubes. The bronchioles also lined with mucous membranes for trapping off dust and germs from the air.

- **Pulmonary Alveoli** – tiny air sacs outlined by a single-layer membrane in contact with blood capillaries.

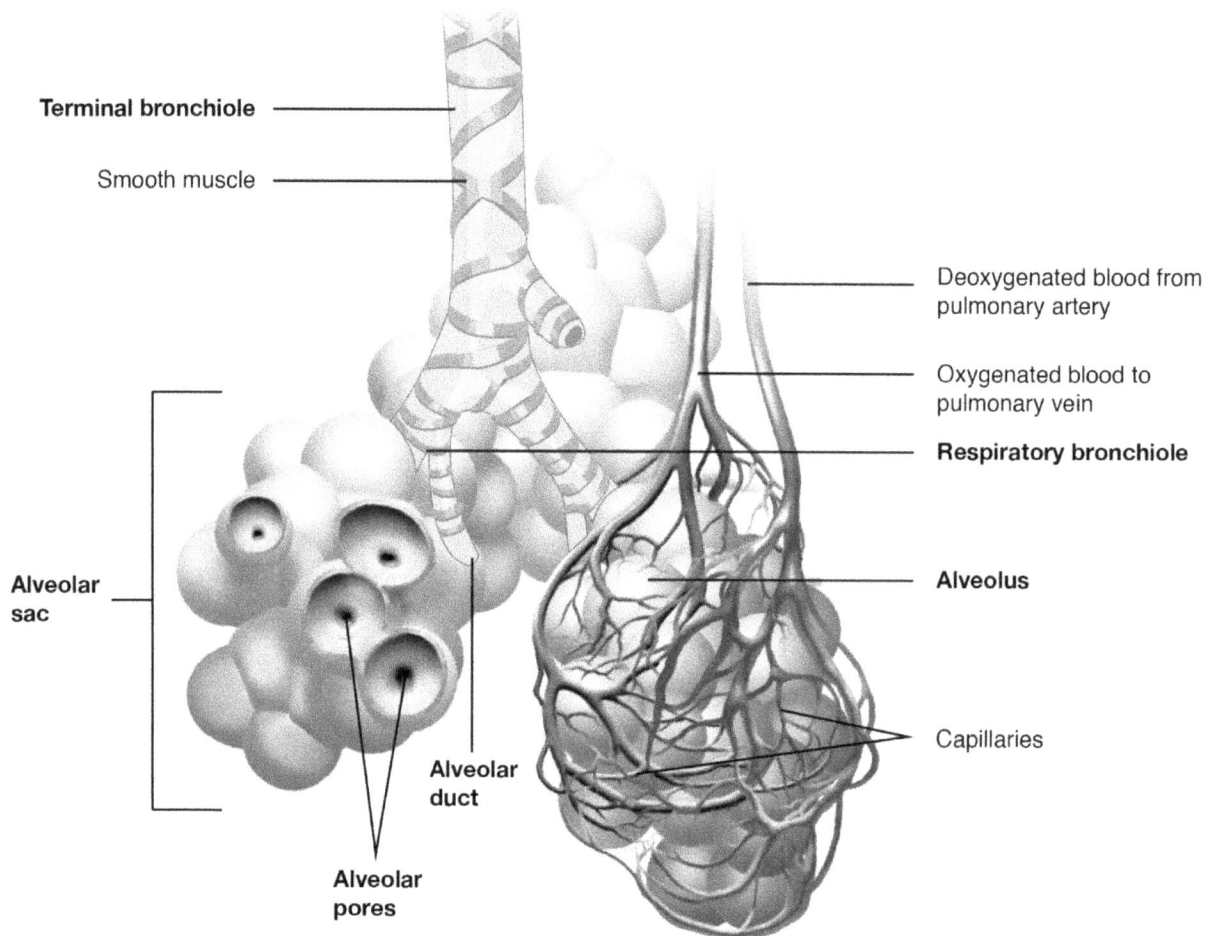

Figure 1-6 Illustration of alveolar structure from Anatomy & Physiology, Connections Web site. http://cnx.org/content/col11496/1.6/ , author: OpenStax College. From Wikimedia Commons.

The exchange of gasses takes place through the membrane of the pulmonary alveolus, which always contains air. Oxygen (O_2) absorbed from the air into the blood capillaries, oxygen binds to hemoglobin as the heart pumps oxygen-binding hemoglobin through all the tissues in the body. At the same time, carbon dioxide (CO_2) is diffused from the blood capillaries into the alveoli, thereby, expelled through the bronchi and the upper respiratory tract.

The lungs' inner surface (as the exchange of gasses takes place) is large because of the structure of the alveolar air sacs.

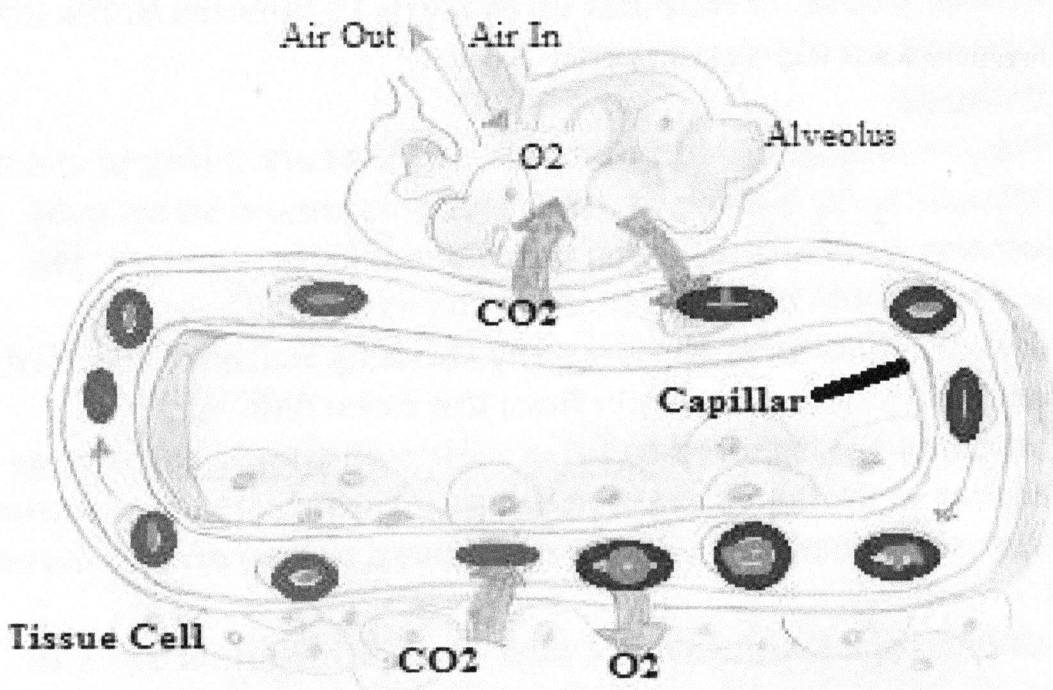

Figure 1-7 illustration of gaseous exchange in the alveoli. O2 from the air is moved into the blood capillary and to the tissues; CO2 is returned from the tissues as the waste product into the capillary and then into the alveoli for exhalation.

The diaphragm is the principal muscle of respiratory system that contracts and relaxes to allow air into the lungs. The structure of diaphragm is a dome-shaped, muscular partition separating the thorax from the abdomen. Contraction and retraction of the diaphragm will increase or decrease the volume of the chest thus inflating and deflating the lungs.

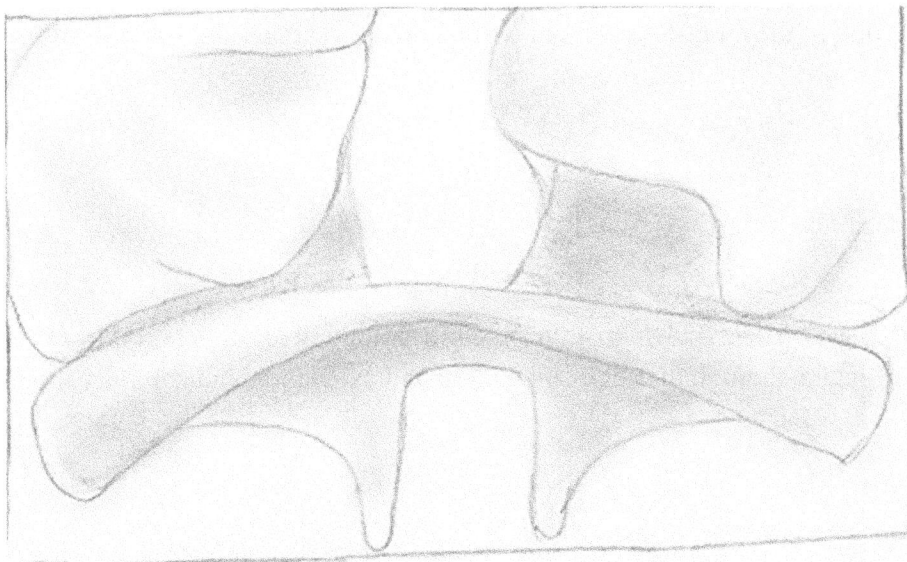

Figure 1-8 displays the anatomy of diaphragm

The act of breathing has two stages known as inhalation and exhalation

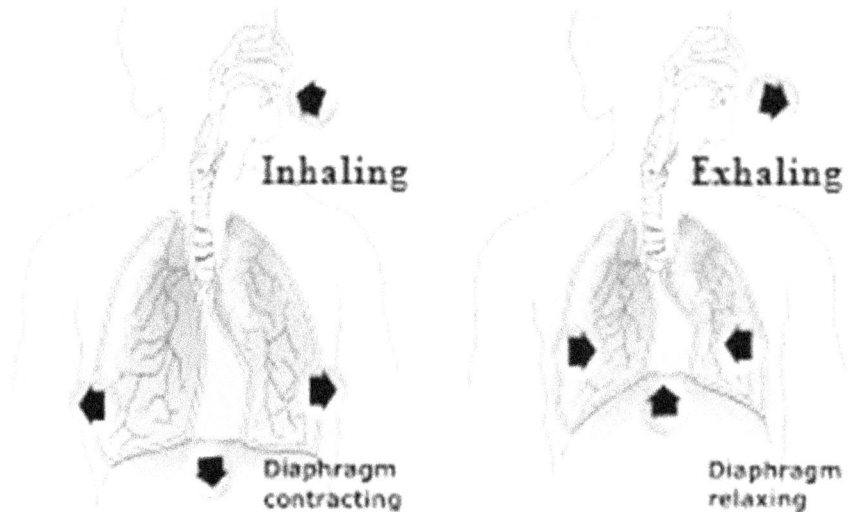

Figure 1-9 shows the inhalation and exhalation mechanism

- The downward motion of the diaphragm results in the increased volume of the chest, causing the lungs to expand sucking in air as it is called breathing in - **inhalation.**

- The upward motion of the diaphragm results in decrease volume of the chest causing contraction of the lungs to expel out air known as breathing out - **exhalation.**

Physiology of Breathing

The figure 1-10, shown below, demonstrates the physiology of air circulation from the atmospheric air intake through the act of inhalation and exhalation and capillary blood flow to the tissues.

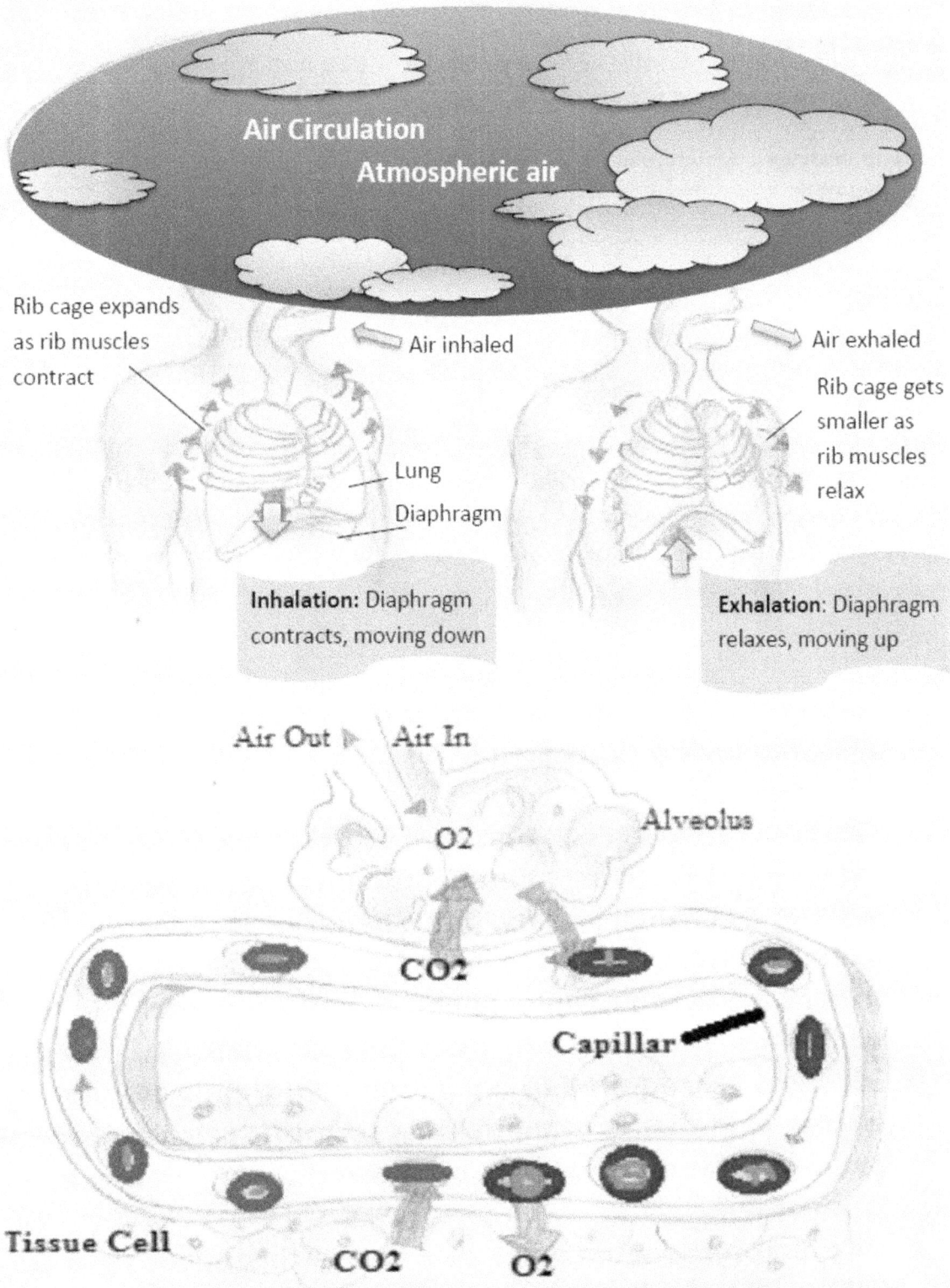

Figure 1-10. Illustration of the physiology of air circulation through the respiratory system and exchange of O2 and CO2 through capillary blood flow to the tissues.

Inhalation and exhalation involve **accessory muscles of Respiratory System**

- **Rib muscles** are intercostal muscles that run between the ribs and help form and move the chest wall.

- **Diaphragm muscle**

The **rib muscles** and **diaphragm** are in constant contraction and relaxation (approximately 12 to 20 times/minute), thus causing the thoracic cavity to rise and fall. Surrounding the lungs are sets of muscles that enable inhalation and exhalation of air from the lungs.
The diaphragm identified as the major muscle of respiration in the human body. The diaphragm is a thin sheet of skeletal muscle that shapes the base of the thorax. The contraction of the diaphragm moves the muscle inferiorly a few inches into the abdominal cavity, expanding space within the thoracic cavity thus drawing air into the lungs. Conversely, as the diaphragm relaxes, air is forced and exhaled out of the lungs.

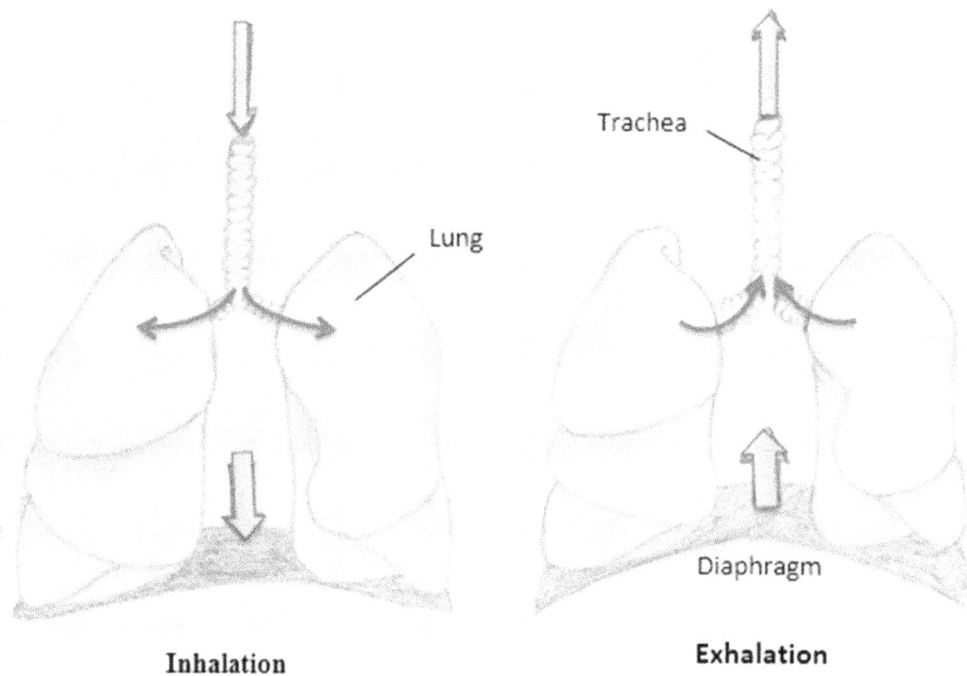

Figure 1-11 displays the function of diaphragm in breathing

Intercostal muscles between the ribs assist the diaphragm with expanding and compressing the lungs. These muscles divided into two groups:

- **Internal Intercostal Muscles**
- **External Intercostal Muscles**

The **internal intercostal muscles** are considered exhalation muscles. As a deeper set of muscles, they depress the ribs to compress the thoracic cavity, causing decrease space in the thoracic cavity resulting air to be exhaled from the lungs.

The **external intercostal muscles** are found superficial to the internal intercostal muscles and function to raise the ribs thereby expanding the volume of the thoracic cavity and causing air to be inhaled into the lungs.

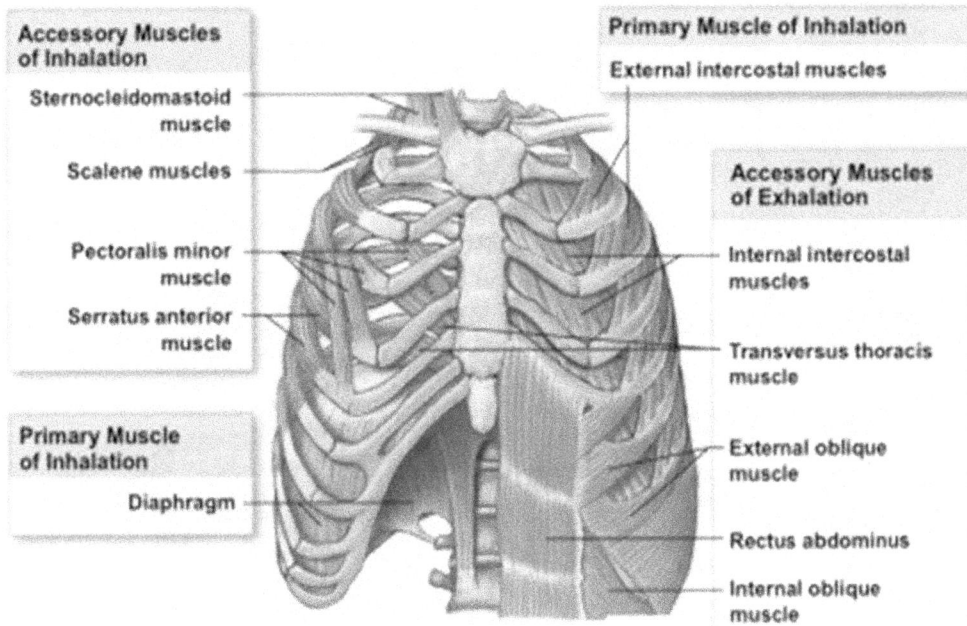

Figure 1-12 Displays the anterior view of primary and accessory respiratory muscles at rest.

During inhalation – the muscles contract:
- Contraction of the diaphragm muscle causes the diaphragm to flatten, thus enlarging the chest cavity and increasing the volume of the thoracic cavity.
- Contraction of the intercostal muscles causes the ribs to elevate, thus increasing the chest volume.

The combination of Diaphragm and rib muscle functions causes the internal pressure in the lungs to be lower than the atmospheric pressure. The thoracic cavity expands, hence reducing air pressure as well as causing air to be passively drawn into the lungs. Air permits from the higher pressure outside the lungs to the inferior pressure inside the lungs. The difference in pressure forces air and introduces oxygen to the alveoli in the lungs.

During exhalation – the muscles relax
The diaphragm arcs and rises, the ribs descend, and chest volume decreases.
The rib cage unwinds to its usual position, and the diaphragm pushes upwards reducing the volume of the thoracic cavity. Therefore, the internal pressure in the lungs becomes greater than the atmospheric pressure. Thus, the difference in pressure forces air out of the lungs expelling carbon dioxide.

The act of breathing – Illustration & Animation

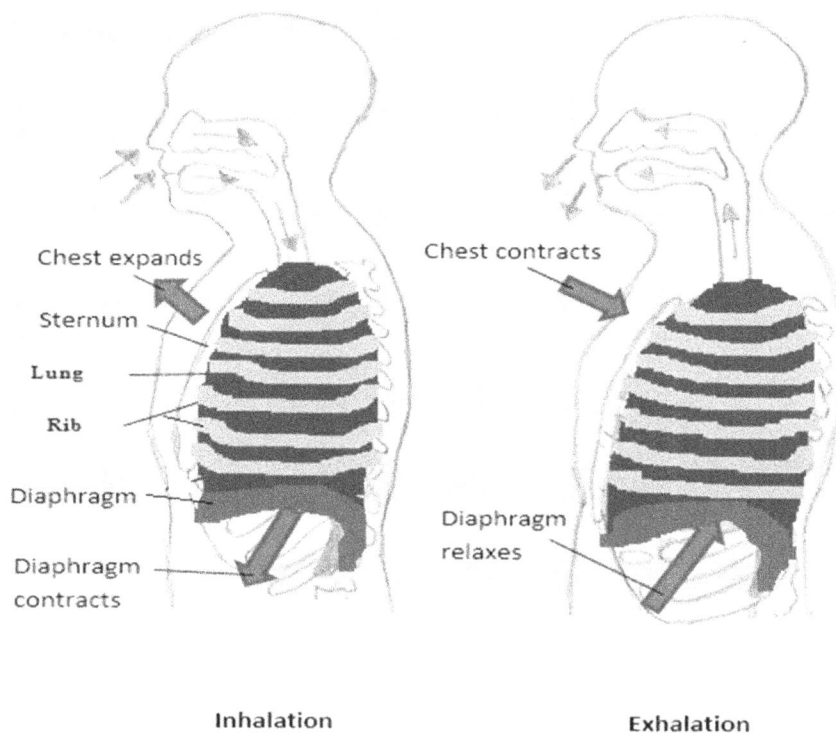

Figure 1-13 illustrates the mechanism of breathing

Variations in chest volume during inhalation and exhalation – requires only the movement of the diaphragm, not that of the rib muscles.

Movement of Oxygen and Carbon Dioxide In and Out of the Respiratory System

```
[Oxygen-rich air from environment] → [Nasal cavities] → [Pharynx] → [Trachea] → [Bronchi]
                                                                                      ↓
[Bronchi] ← [Bronchioles] ← [Oxygen and carbon dioxide exchange at alveoli] ← [Alveoli] ← [Bronchioles]
   ↓
[Trachea] → [Pharynx] → [Nasal cavities] → [Carbon dioxide-rich air to the environment]
```

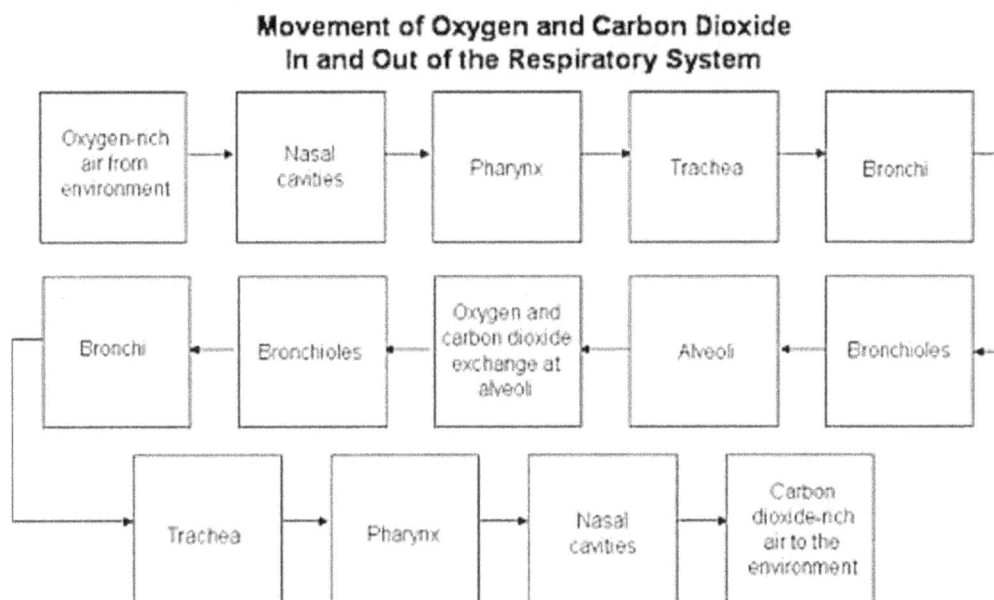

Figure 1-14 Illustrates the respiratory pathways of O2 and CO2 exchange.

The cells and the tissues of the human body necessitate a constant stream of oxygen to stay alive. The respiratory system provides oxygen (O_2) as well as the removal of carbon dioxide (CO_2), a waste product that can be fatal if permitted to accumulate. The respiratory system composed of three major parts: the airway, the lungs, and the muscles of respiration as well as many minor parts.

Oxygen enters the lungs through the nose or the mouth. However, it is best that oxygen enters through the external nares because the nasal hair filters out unwanted substances, warms and humidifies the air. Preferably, the oxygen moves in through the external nares and then passes through the nasal cavity as well as internal nares to reach the nasopharynx. The nasopharynx lies above the point of food entry into the pharynx that is a passageway for air only. From the nasopharynx, oxygen transfers through the oropharynx and the laryngopharynx to reach the larynx. The larynx attached to the hyoid bone superiorly and the trachea inferiorly; it provides an opening to the airway that allows production of many of the sounds associated with voice. From the larynx air travels to the trachea, also known as the windpipe; this begins just inferior to the larynx in the cervical region. As the air moves through the larynx it passes into the chest cavity where the trachea splits at the carina into two smaller tubes called the bronchi; these bronchial tubes then lead the air directly into the lungs. When reaches the lungs, the tubes divide into smaller tubes known as bronchiole that connect the air to alveoli. Alveoli are tiny, balloon-shape sacs at the terminal end of the bronchial tree in the lungs.The exchange of gas (oxygen, O_2, and carbon dioxide, CO_2) takes place in the alveoli. Oxygen from the inhaled air diffuses through the walls of the alveoli and absorbed into adjacent capillaries and the red blood cells in the bloodstream by pulmonary veins. Thus, the oxygen is distributed by the blood to the tissues of the body. Through the action of body's metabolism, carbon dioxide (CO_2) produced that returns to the lung through the blood. As a waste product of the lungs from the pulmonary artery, CO_2 diffuses through the capillary blood flow and alveolar walls into the air to be eliminated from the body with expiration.

Oxygen transport

Oxygen carried in two forms in the blood:

• Oxygen molecules combined with hemoglobin (97%).Hemoglobin molecule consists of two alpha and two beta chains; each chain is formed from an iron–porphyrin molecule called "haem." Each hemoglobin molecule can bind by four oxygen molecules that are 20 mL oxygen per 100mL of blood or 15mL oxygen per 100mL in venous blood.

• Oxygen dissolved in the blood accounts for a minimal amount (0.3 mL/dL); the volume dissolved comply with Henrys' law that is proportional to the partial pressure 0.023mL per KPa per 100mL of blood.

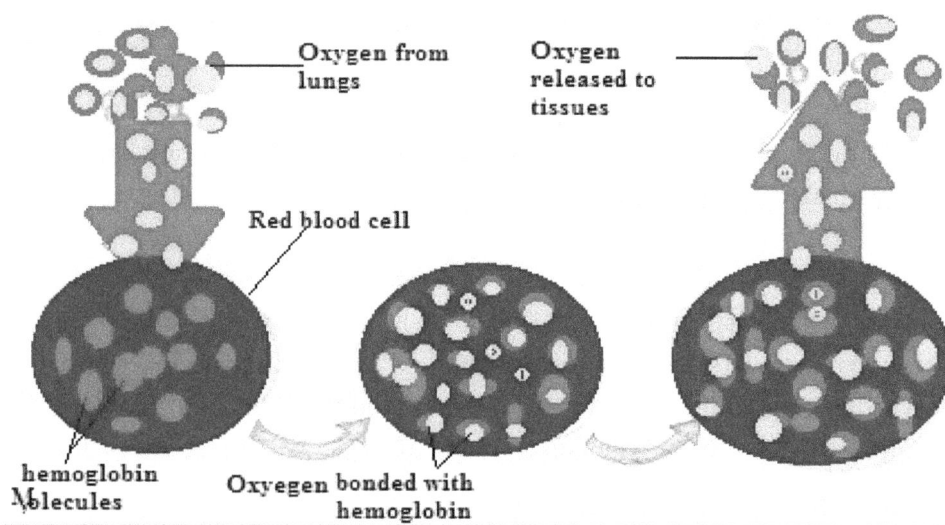

Figure 1-15 shows the oxygen transport from the lungs to red blood cell binding to hemoglobin molecules and released to the tissue cells.

Blood Oxygen Content

Total content of oxygen in the blood calculated from the Oxygen flux equation:

Flux = [(CO X Hb X SaO_2 X 1.39 (Haffner's constant) + (0.003 X PaO_2)].

Oxygen-Dissociation-Curve

- Sigmoid shaped curve concerning the fact that binding of oxygen to the hemoglobin molecule is a cooperative process
- Describes the relationship of saturation of hemoglobin with oxygen at fluctuating partial pressures
- Be aware of the P50 that is a point at which Hb is 50% saturated
- Declining pH, the rise in temperature, 2,3-DPG, and CO_2 tension causes the curve to shift to the right.
- Rise of pH and fall in CO2 tension, temperature, and 2,3-DPG causes the curve to shift to the left
- If the curve shift to the right the hemoglobin (Hb) molecule has higher probability to unload oxygen (O_2) to the tissues
- In a left shifted circumstances, the hemoglobin (Hb) is less liable to release oxygen to the tissues

Oxygen dissociation curve of adult hemoglobin

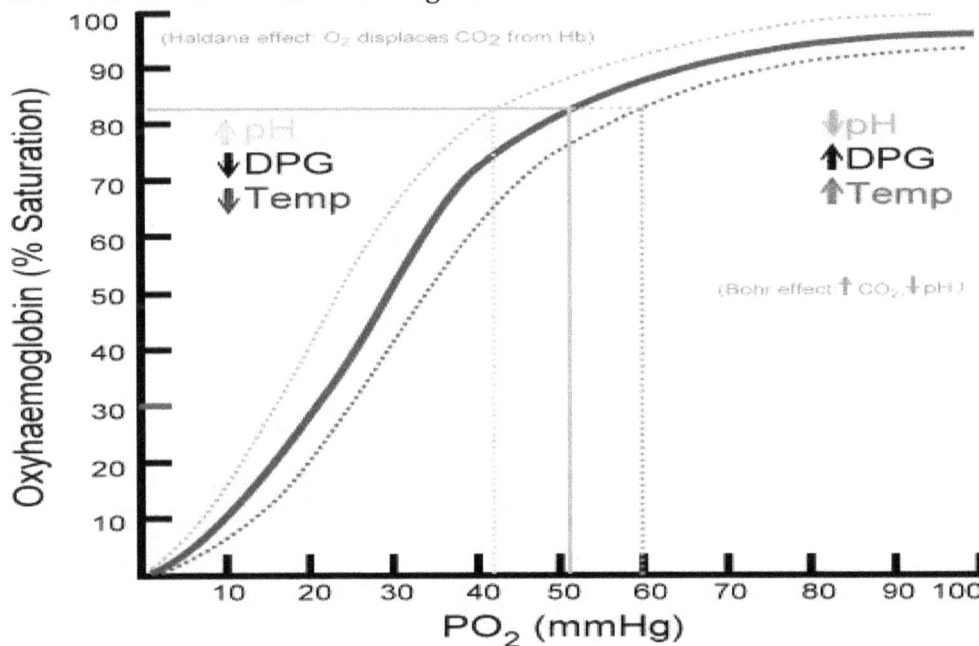

2,3-DPG

This molecule binds to deoxygenated hemoglobin as it reduces the affinity of hemoglobin for oxygen and, therefore, confirms unloading of oxygen to the tissues.

The Bohr Effect

Describes the CO_2 influencing the release of oxygen to the tissues. Upon entering red blood cells, the following reaction occurs:

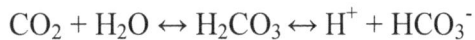

$$CO_2 + H_2O \leftrightarrow H_2CO_3 \leftrightarrow H^+ + HCO_3^-$$

An increase in H^+ will cause an acidosis, therefore, results in encouraging the release of oxygen from Hb. Moreover, In the lungs where the CO_2 is being removed, the alkalosis will encourage the uptake of oxygen.

Oxygen Delivery (DO_2)

Calculated as follows:
DO_2 = Cardiac Output X Arterial O_2 Content
DO_2 = CO X CaO_2

Carbon dioxide transport

The three ways that carbon dioxide (CO_2) carried in the blood are:

- As bicarbonate – 90%
- As dissolved CO_2 – 5%
- As carbamino compounds – 5%

Carbamino compounds shaped by the response of the CO_2 with terminal amino groups of proteins and side chains of arginine and lysine. Hemoglobin is essential for this process to occur since it has four amino groups per molecule. Also, albumin provides amino groups but only 1 per molecule.

The Haldane effect

It refers to the increased ability of blood to carry CO_2 when hemoglobin is deoxygenated. Deoxyhemoglobin is 3.5 times more efficient than oxyhemoglobin in forming carbamino compound.

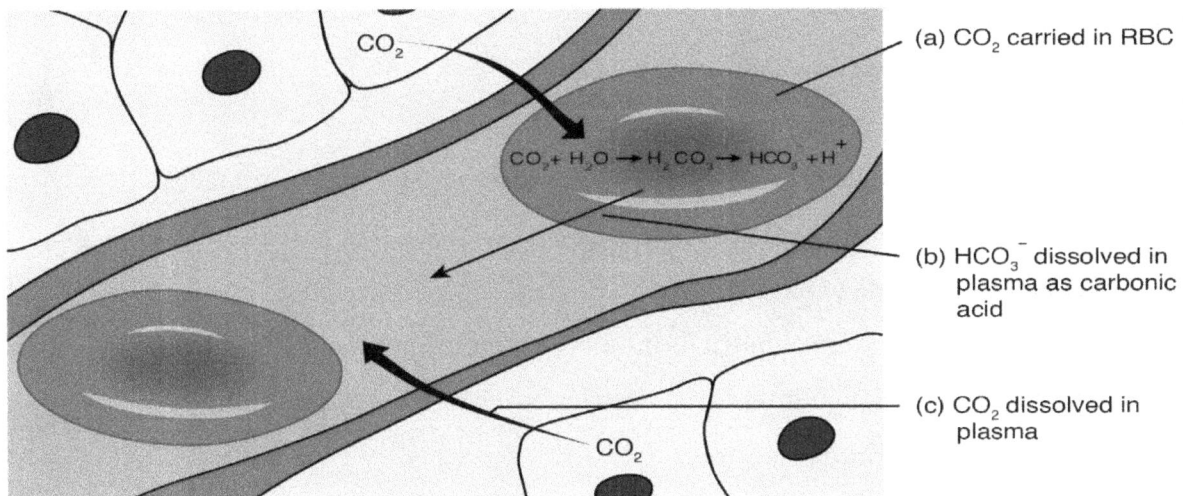

Figure 1-17 Illustration of carbon dioxide transport in blood by OpenStack College-Anatomy and Physiology, Connection website, http://cnx.org/content/col11496/1.6/, Jan 19, 2013. Vectorized by Kaidor, CC BY-SA 3.0, https://commons.wikimedia.org/w/index.php?curid=34138672.

1. Explain the process of producing energy.
2. Explain the aerobic respiration equation.
3. Explain the two primary elements of the respiratory system, the upper respiratory tract and lower respiratory tract.
4. Explain the process of gas exchange.
5. Describe the two stages known as inhalation and exhalation.
6. Explain the function of intercostal muscles in the process of breathing.
7. Explain the respiratory pathways.
8. Describe Oxygen-Dissociation-Curve.
9. What is The Bohr Effect?
10. Explain the Haldane effect.

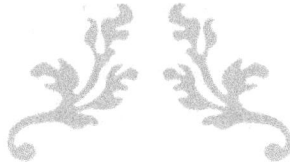

Chapter 2

Respiratory Assessment and Diagnostic Procedures

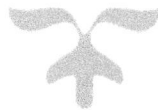

Chapter Objectives

1. Describe the life functions
2. Perform the chest assessment
3. Explain the Ventilatory-Perfusion ratio
4. Define the Ventilatory Regulation
5. Explain the mechanism of Pulmonary Shunt
6. Explain the lung compliance
7. Describe airway resistance
8. Explain the cough and sputum production
9. Describe Polycythemia, Core-Pulmonale
10. Explain the Arterial Blood Gasses and its process
11. Explain the Pulmonary Function Test (PFT) and its process
12. Explain the Electrocardiogram (ECG, EKG)

Life Functions are the process of getting air and oxygen from the outside environment, through the lungs, into the blood, and to the tissues. The four critical life functions are:

- **Ventilation** involves breathing air into and out of the lung. It is the initial assessment step in assuring patent airway and proper air movement for adequate ventilation.

- **Oxygenation** is a process of getting an appropriate amount of oxygen into the blood as evaluated by heart rate, color, and sensorium.

- **Circulation** is moving blood through the body as assessed by pulse strength, regularity, and cardiac output.

- **Perfusion** is getting blood and oxygen into the tissue by evaluating adequate blood pressure, color and sensorium, known as the fourth step in the life function process.

Lungs are altered to an extent when they exposed to certain disease or trauma. The classification of theses alterations includes an Obstructive, Restrictive or combination of both, (Obstructive and Restrictive lung disease). Table 2-1 below lists common respiratory disorders based on their classification.

TABLE 2-1 Classification of Respiratory Disorders

Obstructive	Restrictive	Combination
Asthma	Pneumonia	Bronchiectasis[*]
Chronic Bronchitis	Pulmonary edema	Cystic Fibrosis[*]
Emphysema	ARDS	Pneumoconiosis
	Flail Chest	
	Pneumothorax	
	Pleural disease	
	Kyphoscoliosis	
	Tuberculosis	
	Fungal Disease	
	IRDS	
*most commonly seen as an obstructive pulmonary disease		

The modification of the normal anatomy of the lung causes pathophysiologic mechanisms of the pulmonary system to occur. These pathophysiologic mechanisms lead to numerous clinical signs such as increased heart rate, hypoventilation, hyperventilation, high functional residual capacity, and other clinical manifestations. Therefore, healthcare professionals must have the familiarity of the abnormality in the anatomic state of the lungs as emerged by the disease, pathophysiologic mechanisms triggered by illness and clinical signs associated with the disorder. In doing so, the health care provider should examine a general physical examination of the chest as a first step in the process.

Assessment of the Chest

The physical examination and chest inspection performed in a systematic and consistent method. The order for this procedure is as follows:

1. Inspection (observe)
2. Palpation (Feel)
3. Percussion (Tap)
4. Auscultation (Listen)

Chest Inspection

Chest inspection can provide an enormous amount of essential data for the healthcare provider to identify the existence and lack of certain clinical features. The medical personnel should pay significant attention to the following areas:

Table 2-2 displays the chest inspection

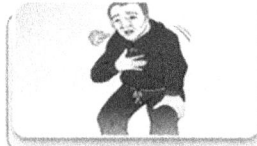

Shortness of Breath (SOB)
- Does the patient pause to breathe while speaking?

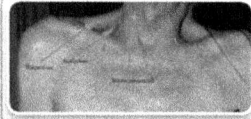

Accessory muscle
- Does Patient use accessory muscle during inspiration and expiration?

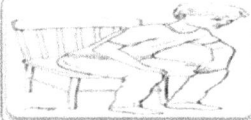

Posture:
- Does patient lean forward, hold on to an object, and bending their shoulder forward?

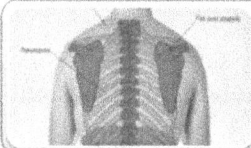

Symmetry
Is the patient's chest, scapulae symmetric and spine straight?

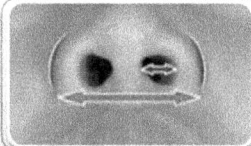

Nasal flaring:
Does patient have nasal flaring during inspiration and expiration?

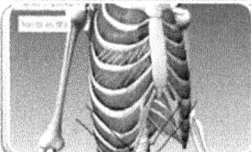

Intercostal space retraction:
Does patient have intercostal space retraction during inspiration?

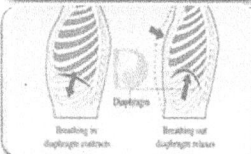

Ventilatory Pattern:
Patient's respiratory rate and depth of breathing.

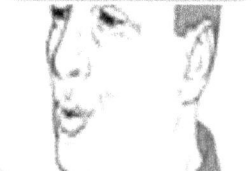

Pursed Lip breathing:
Does patient display pursed lip breathing during ventilation.

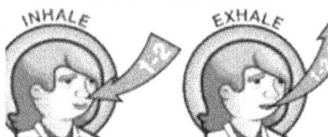

I:E Ratio:
Patient's inspiratory to expiratory ratio.

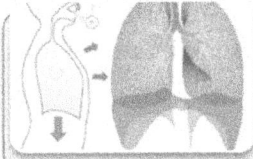

Excursion of the Chest Wall

Does the patients diaphragm move downward during inspiration?

Does thoracic cage move upward and outward during inspiration?

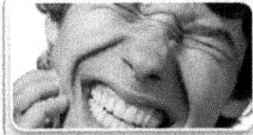

Splinting

is patient splinting to control pain? It might be suggestive of rib fracture, pneumonia, pneumothorax, pleural effusion and postoperative pain.

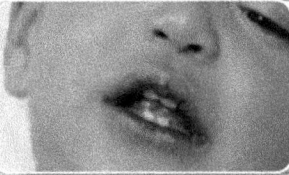

Skin Condition and Color

Is patient cyanotic or perhaps dehydrated?

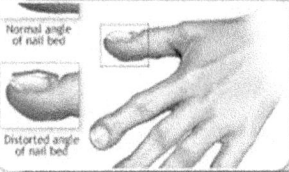

Hand and Nail-beds

are hands and nails show sign of cyanosis and digital clubbing?

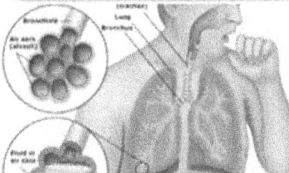

Cough

Is patient coughing? if yes, then what type of cough is produced by patient?

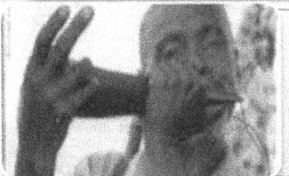

Audible Wheezing or Rhonchi

Is there audible wheezing sound and rhonchi while patient is breathing?

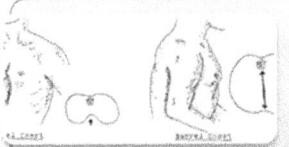

Barrel Chest(increased A-P diameter)

Does patient have barrel chest?

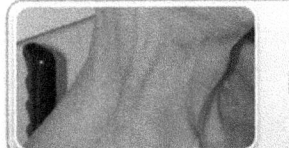

Edema and Distended Neck Veins

is there indication of edema and distended neck or face veins? this may suggest CHF(congestive heart failure)

Variances in breathing forms can give hints to ailments of multiple diverse organ systems as much as the respiratory system alone. The pattern of breathing encompasses the rate, rhythm, and volume of a patient's breathing. The regular breathing rate is 12-20 breaths per minute, with an approximate 1:4 ratio of inhalation to exhalation.

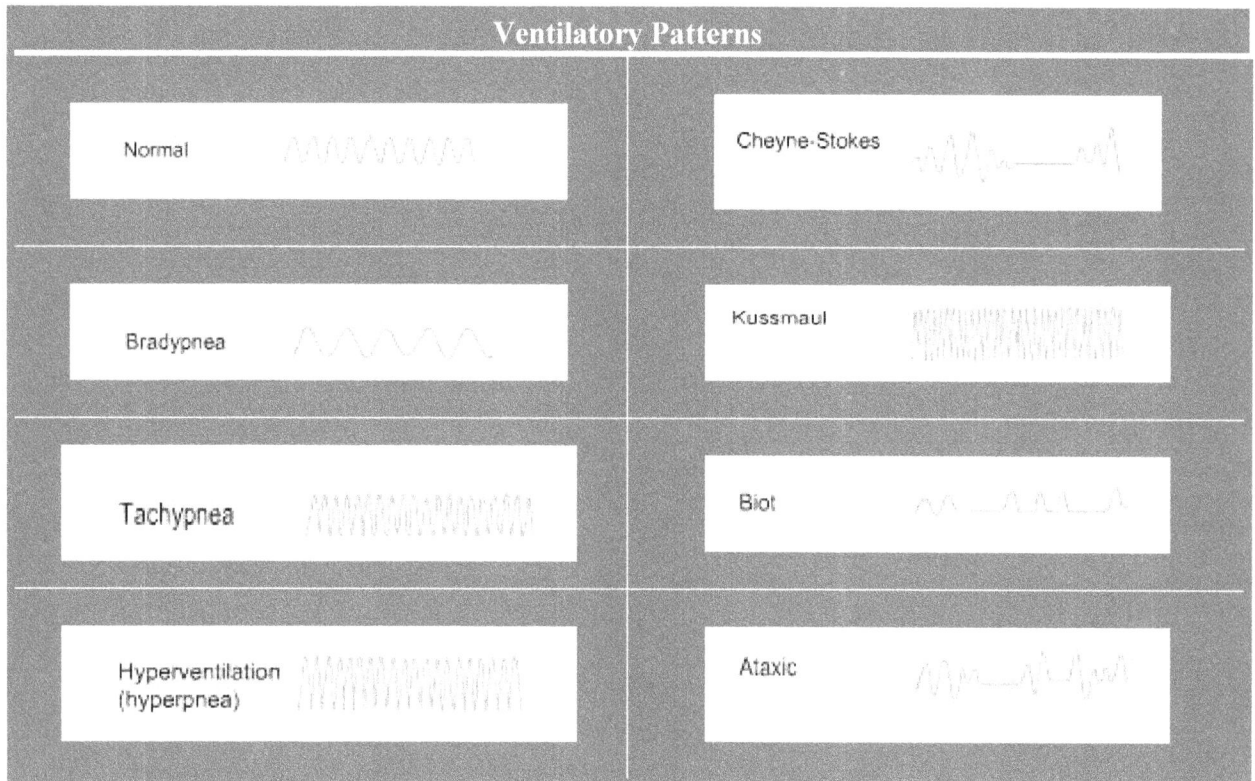

Figure 2-1 shows the variation of breathing patterns

Three key abnormal breathing patterns described as follows:

- Cheyne-Stokes respiration described by episodes of apnea that scattered between cycles of gradually increasing then decreasing respiratory rates, that often specifies uremia or congestive heart failure (CHF).
- Kussmaul breathing is a fast, large-volume breathing produced by acidotic stimulation of the respiratory center; it can point toward metabolic acidosis.
- Biot breathing is an uneven breathing pattern alternating among tachypnea, bradypnea, and apnea, a potential sign of impending respiratory failure.

Palpation

Palpation is the process of palpable examination of the chest to evaluate:

- Tenderness - Local tenderness points to trauma or costochondritis.

- Asymmetry and diaphragmatic excursion - Evaluated by placing one hand posteriorly on each hemithorax close to the diaphragm level with the palms facing anteriorly and thumbs touching at the midline. When the patient inhales, each hand should rotate away from the midline alike. Uneven movement, or a small movement, specifies asymmetry and poor diaphragmatic excursion, correspondingly.

- Crepitus - Crepitus is the feeling of crackles under the fingertips during external palpation of the chest wall indicating the presence of subcutaneous air often linked with a pneumothorax on the side of the abnormality.

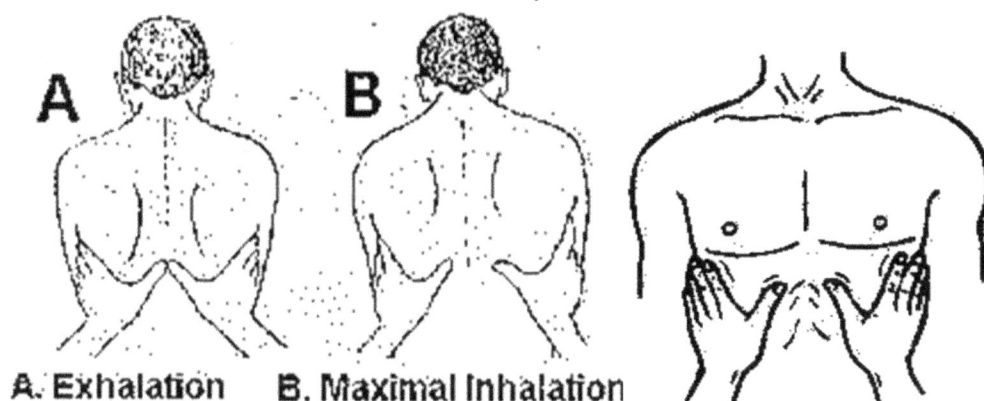

Figure 2-2 displays tactile examination of the chest

- Vocal fremitus - After external palpation, a profound review of the lungs and air spaces can be accomplished through testing for vocal fremitus. The assessor places the ulnar edge of the hand on the chest wall while the patient echoes a particular slogan, usually "ninety-nine" (99) or "one, two, three." (1, 2,3) The strength of the vibrations felt designates the attenuation of sounds transferred through the lung tissues. Regions of amplified vibration or fremitus relate to areas of increased density of the tissue such as those caused by consolidation, pneumonia or malignancy. Superimposing fatty tissue increased airspace as evident by COPD, or fluid-filled lung space may decrease perceived fremitus.

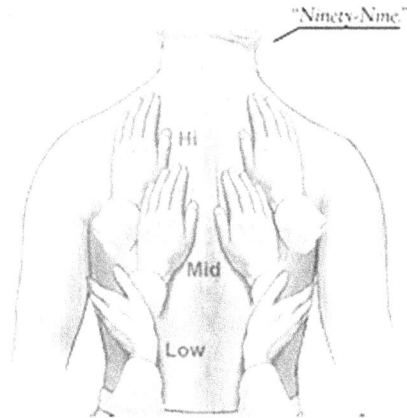

Figure 2-3 shows the Vocal fremitus examination of the chest and hand placement as "Hi, Mid, and Low position.

Percussion

Percussion of the chest is performed to obtain information regarding the presence of air or consolidation within the chest cavity. Percussion accomplished by placing the pad of the nondominant middle finger on the chest wall no other part of the hand should be in contact with touch the patient. The tip of the dominant middle finger is used to strike the distal interphalangeal joint of the positioned finger. This procedure should be applied to the regions shown in the images below, equating the two hemithoraces.

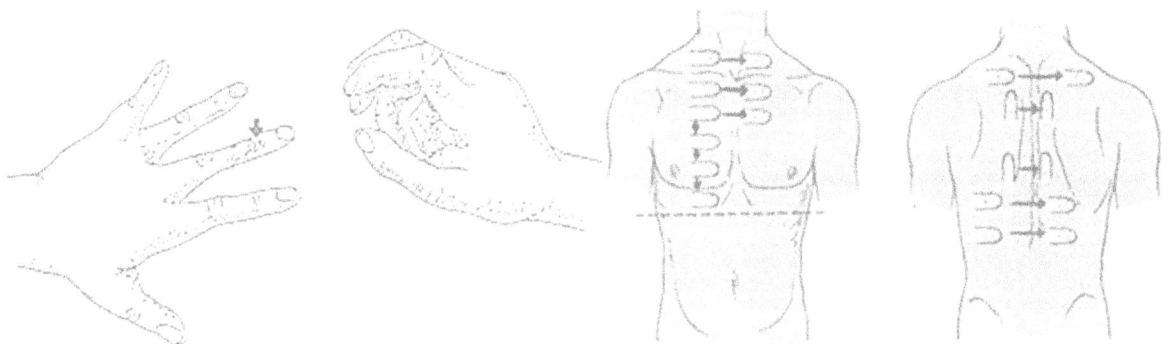

Figure 2-4 Illustrates the percussion method and finger placement on the chest

Percussion creates sounds on a scale from flat to dull contingent on the density of the underlying tissue. Areas of the well-aerated lung referred to as resonant sound, or tympanic, to percussion.

Abnormal percussion sound is Dull percussion note and Hyperresonant percussion note. Dullness to percussion specifies denser tissue, such as areas of effusion or consolidation. The sounds produced usually described as dull, soft in pitch and short in duration same as generated by knocking on a full barrel.

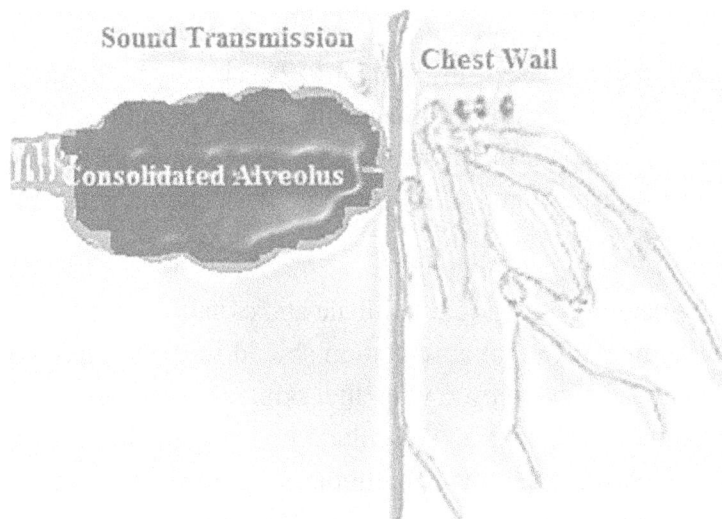

Figure 2-5 shows dull percussion note produced over zone of effusion or consolidation

Hyperresonant note produced over areas of trapped gas. These sounds are deafening, low in pitch and long in duration suggestive of knocking on an empty barrel. Hyperresonant notes commonly elicited in patients with the chronic obstructive pulmonary disease and pneumothorax. Upon detection of an abnormality, percussion can be used around the area of concern to define the magnitude of the abnormality.

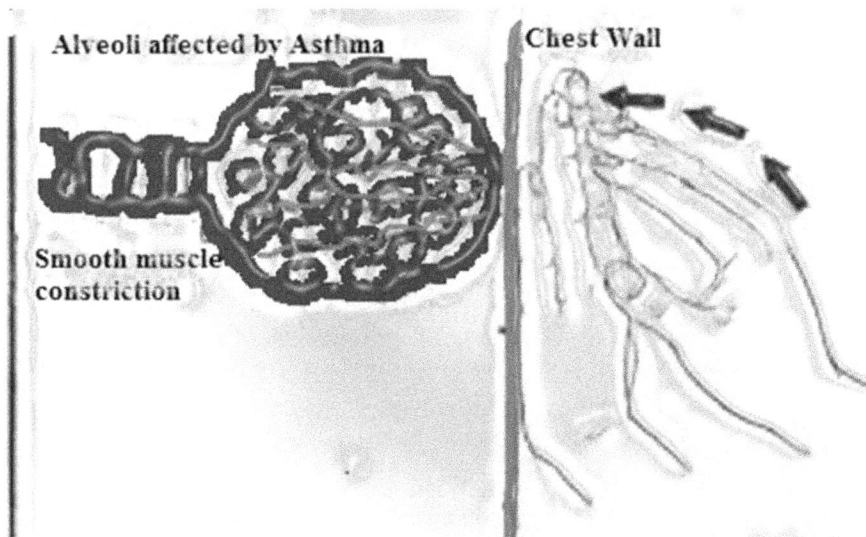

Figure 2-6 Display of hyper-resonant sound over Hyperinflated alveoli

Typical zones of dullness are those covering the liver and spleen at the anterior bases of the lungs. Normal regions of tympany cover the gastric bubble, often obscuring the dullness induced by the spleen. As with fremitus, sounds fluctuate subject to the thickness of subcutaneous tissues.

Auscultation

Before auscultation, it is recommended the patient to be placed in a sitting position. In certain situations where a patient is to remain recumbent, the patient should be rolled from one side to the other to auscultate the back. Furthermore, If the patient cannot be turned from side to side, such as in certain intensive care units (ICU) settings, the anterior chest can be auscultated to produce a more limited checkup.

During auscultation, the patient is instructed to inhale and exhale deeper than their normal breaths through the mouth. It is imperative that auscultation should be performed with the diaphragm of the stethoscope to have a direct contact with the skin, as clothing and other materials can diminish or distort perceived lung sounds. Auscultate in a pattern shown in the images below as performed symmetrically between the two hemithoraces, so that sounds paralleled between sides. Start auscultation near the apices and move down in a ladder-like pattern to the lower level of the diaphragm or until the breath sounds are no longer valued. The auscultation should be performed over the anterior and posterior chest.

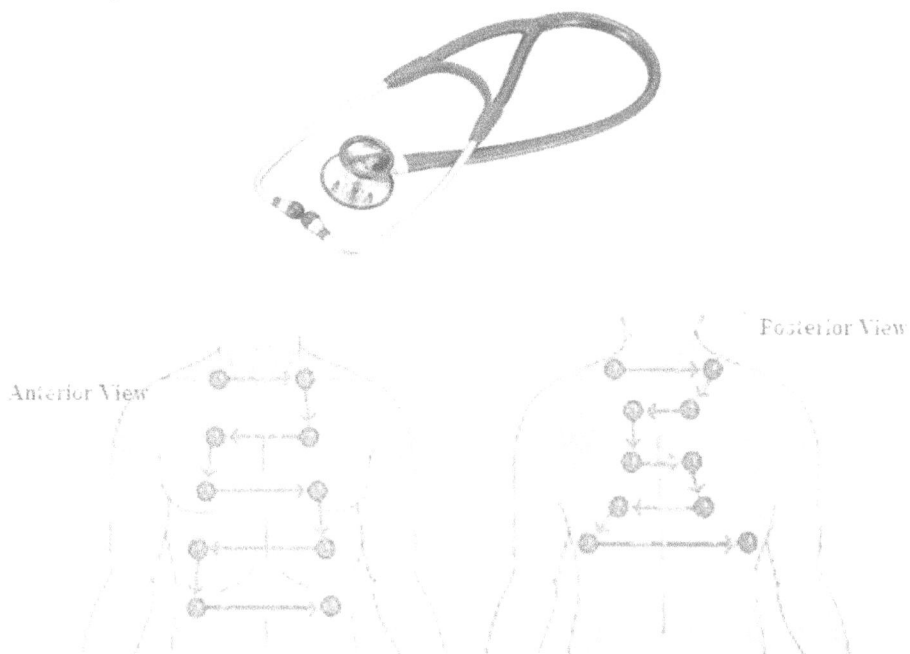

Figure 2-7 Illustrated the auscultation marking of anterior and posterior of the chest

Normal Breath Sounds

The sounds heard during auscultation can be categorized as breath sounds, created by air movement through the airway structures of the tracheobronchial tree. As the rate of flow changes significantly between trachea and alveoli; therefore, the nature and tone of breath-sound change as well.

Auscultation over the trachea and large bronchi has tubular, and bronchial quality since the sound is loud and high pitched that commonly referred to as normal bronchial breath sounds. Bronchial breath sounds are louder during expiration; there is also a pause between the inspiration phase and expiration phase.

Broncho-vesicular or Vesicular Sounds

Vesicular sounds are produced by the turbulent flow of air through the airways of healthy lungs. Over the parenchyma region of normal lungs, the breath sounds are more evident during inspiration, and they are much softer, and lower in pitch that is because gas molecules entering the alveoli distribute out over the larger surface area thereby create less gas turbulence. Consequently, decreased gas turbulence leads to decrease breath sounds. These vesicular sounds diverge significantly from patient to patient; thus, it is essential to listen in a symmetrical pattern to compare one hemidiaphragm to another.

Abnormal Breath Sounds Classified as the following:

- Bronchial breath sounds
- Absent or diminished breath sounds
- Crackles and rhonchi
- Wheeze
- Pleural friction rub
- Whispered pectoriloquy

Bronchial Breath Sounds

Bronchial breath sounds frequently result from consolidation or atelectasis within lung parenchyma with a patent airway leading to the involved zone. The gas molecule has no opportunity to extend over a larger surface area and, therefore, becomes less turbulent.

Consequently, the resulting breath sounds are amplified through the consolidation, leading to a louder breath sound since the gas sound are coming mainly from the tracheobronchial tree, not the lung parenchyma. Normally, between inspiratory and expiratory sounds there is a gap or pause, as the involved parenchyma does not fill with air during this period in inspiration. The tone is usually high, as the sounds arise from the bronchi, and the expiratory phase usually lasts longer and is just as intense, or stronger than, the inspiratory phase.

Absent / Diminished Breath Sounds

Absent or diminished breath sounds occur when there is no airflow or limited airflow to the region being auscultated. Disorders causing hypoventilation such as chronic obstructive pulmonary disease normally have diminished breath sounds. Hypoventilation, in this case, results from air trapping and increased functional residual capacity associated with obstructive lung disorders. Consequently, when the functional residual capacity is elevated so the surface area of the alveoli, therefore, entering gas to these larger than normal area results in less gas turbulence and a softer sound. Diminished breath sounds can occur in a pneumothorax, hemothorax, pleural effusion, flail chest as well as neuromuscular diseases such as Guillain-Barre' syndrome and myasthenia gravis.

Adventitious sounds

Adventitious sounds classified as crackles, wheezes, rhonchi, or stridor. These sounds arise in addition to the breath sounds defined above.

Crackles

Crackles are sounds that are bubbly or slurpy wet, intermittent, nonmusical, and more noticeable during inspiration. The rubbing sound of hair between one's fingers frequently used as an illustration to describe these kinds of sounds. The two classifications of Crackles are fine and coarse crackles, contingent on the quality of their sound that are typically heard at the time of inspiration.

Fine crackles naturally produced by the forced reopening of alveoli that had closed in the course of the past expiration. Fine crackles are characterized by softer and higher in pitch as compared to coarse crackles that are louder and lower in pitch. Moreover, Coarse crackles are typically a mixture of alveolar reopening and bubbling of air through retained secretions in smaller airways.

Crackles are formed in small and medium-size airways and commonly do not change in nature after a vigorous cough.

Rhonchi

Rhonchi are low-pitched, course, bubbly and snore like sounds that typically heard during expiration. Rhonchi are frequently characterized by secretions within the large airways and often change in nature or cannot be heard after a strong or a vigorous cough. Rhonchi can be heard in a broad range of pathologies, in which cause increased secretions, for instance in emphysema, pneumonia, cystic fibrosis, bronchitis, and pulmonary edema.

Wheezes

Wheezes are continuous, high-pitched, whistling, musical, primarily expiratory sounds that produced by air moving through constricted bronchi resulting in quivering and resonance of the bronchial walls. Thus, wheezing is the characteristic sound produced by bronchospasm. Wheezes caused by pathology leading to the narrowing of bronchi, most commonly asthma, bronchitis, and COPD.

Pleural Friction Rub

The substantial additional sound is a pleural rub, which can be appreciated as having a sandpaper like quality and is typically present throughout the respiratory cycle. Inflammation such as pleuritis accompanies a respiratory disorder can cause thickening of the pleural surfaces and resist movement during breathing. Thickening of the pleural surface thereby creates more friction when sliding along one another, produces a particular sound known as a pleural friction rub.

Stridor sound

It is heard during inspiration and characterized by a loud, rough, continuous, high-pitched sound. Strider indicates proximal airway obstruction. The sound produced by turbulent air rolling through a narrowed trachea or larynx and is loudest over the trachea. Strider is commonly a medical emergency and should be recognized early. Diagnoses that may present with stridor include epiglottitis, vocal cord dysfunction, croup, and airway edema possibly as the result of an allergic response or secondary to trauma.

Pectoriloquy / Egophony

Whispered verses known as pectoriloquy that reduces aeration and results in a change of the transmitted pitch sounds, called egophony. Whispered pectoriloquy is a term used to define the unusual clear transmission of the whispered voice of a patient through the stethoscope.

Whispered pectoriloquy provoked by having the patient whisper a repeated phrase such as "one, two, three" or "ninety-nine"). As the whispered sound travels down the tracheobronchial tree, they remain unchanged, but as the sound disperses throughout the large surface area of the alveoli, it diminishes sharply. Thereby, sound through the stethoscope over a normal lung unit as the patient whispers the phrase "one, two, three or ninety-nine"; the sounds are diminished, distant and incomprehensible. However, the transmitted sounds are louder over the area of consolidation. Egophony stimulated by asking the patient say "ee," and the transmitted sound is heard as "aay" over a consolidated area.

Description of other clinical sign of respiratory disorders

Cyanosis

Cyanosis is blue-gray or purplish discoloration of the mucous membranes, fingertips, toes whenever hemoglobin in these regions reduced to at least 5 gm/dl. Most often cyanosis is seen in severe respiratory diseases. Full saturation of 14-15 gm/dl of hemoglobin yields Pao_2 of about 97-100 mmHg and approximately 20 vol percent of oxygen in the blood. Therefore, patients with cyanosis that have 5 gm/dl of reduced hemoglobin will have a Pao_2 of about 30 mmHg and 13 vol percent of oxygen in the blood. Cyanosis is seen in the skin, nail beds, or mucous membranes.

There are two major types of cyanosis known as:
- **Peripheral (acrocyanosis)**

- **Central cyanosis**.

Peripheral or acrocyanosis is seen only in the limbs that are common in young infants that are a part of normal physiology.

Central cyanosis affects the entire body and well observed in the mucous membranes of the mouth and the tongue. This sign usually means a potentially severe and life-threatening disease and almost always a sign of hypoxemia with a positive diagnostic and prognostic value that requires immediate evaluation. The underlying disease of respiratory origin indicated by a sign of shortness of breath (SOB), rapid breathing, bluish or purple discoloration of the fingers and toes and mouth mucous membranes.

Cyanosis may impact some of the major organs and systems of the body include the respiratory system, cardiovascular system, heart, blood, and the central nervous system (CNS).

In respiratory disorder cyanosis is caused by three leading causes:

1. Decrease ventilation-perfusion ratio ($\dot{V}/\dot{Q}$)
2. Pulmonary Shunting
3. Venous admixture

Ventilation-Perfusion Ratio ($\dot{V}/\dot{Q}$)

The ventilation-perfusion (V/Q) ratio describes the dynamic relationship between the volume of ventilation in the alveoli and the perfusion amount through the alveolar capillaries. This association determines the quality of gas exchange across the alveolar–capillary membrane, which in turn controls the volume of oxygen inflowing the blood and unloading of CO_2 from the blood. Consequently, the utilization of this relationship describes the etiology of hypoxemia. Within the normal lung, each alveolus would receive an adequate volume of ventilation and similar measurements of blood flow through the adjacent capillary, resulting in a V/Q ratio of "1" indicating that ventilation and perfusion are equal. This perfect situation never exists, due to the effects of gravity on the flow of blood, the lungs structure, and the blood shunting. For example in a standing position, the lungs pull downward due to gravity toward the diaphragm, thereby, compressing the lower lobes, and the flow of blood pulled to the lungs bases. Moreover, air moves upward to the apexes of the lungs and increases the residual volume. Apexes of the lungs are larger and have a higher surface tension, but they are fewer in number compared with other regions of the lungs. The lungs apexes with larger alveoli have a higher surface tension that reduces their compliant and harder to inflate during ventilation. Consequently, the tidal volume shifted to a more compliant space such as the lower lobes, where there is less surface tension.

As gravity pulls the blood downward, less pressure is necessary to perfuse the inferior lobes of the lungs, as paralleled with the apexes, which are above the level of the heart. Furthermore, the greatest volume of ventilation also exists in the lung base. The $\dot{V}/\dot{Q}$ ratio is under no circumstances at an idyllic state in any areas of the lungs. In the lungs apexes, the amount of available ventilation in the alveoli surpasses the volume of perfusion through the pulmonary capillaries; while more oxygen is present in the alveoli than the supply of blood can collect and transport, this phenomenon known as wasted ventilation. In the bases of the lungs, the amount of perfusion tops the amount of ventilation that considered being dead space or wasted perfusion. Overall, under normal circumstances, perfusion surpasses the amount of available ventilation.

Ventilatory Disturbances

A disruption on the ventilation part of the ventilation-perfusion ratio ($\dot{V}/\dot{Q}$) leads to hypoxia. If a disorder or injury reduces the availability of oxygenated air in the alveoli for the volume of blood moving through the pulmonary capillaries, resulting in lower blood saturation of oxygen as well as a reduction in delivery of oxygen to the cells, producing hypoxemia and cellular hypoxia. For example, during an asthma spell with the inflammation of bronchioles and airway constriction, airflow is reduced and supply a reduced amount of oxygenated air to the alveoli for gas exchange. However, the blood pressure is not affected; therefore, the volume of blood moving through the pulmonary capillaries remains normal. Thereby, a ventilation disturbance has been generated by creating fewer oxygen molecules available to the blood passing through the pulmonary capillaries resulting in a condition known as wasted perfusion; that is in the presence of availability of sufficient volume of blood there is an inadequacy of oxygen to be picked up. Wasted perfusion and disruption in ventilation lead to hypoxemia and cellular hypoxia. In the described situation, in which an asthma attack caused a ventilatory interruption, the ventilation side of the ventilation-perfusion ratio vital to be improved by relieving the bronchiole airway restriction and increasing the sum of the rich oxygenated air flowing into the alveoli.

Hypoxia is commonly due to ventilation or perfusion disruption. Numerous conditions can cause one of these disturbances to occur. Enhancing oxygenation and ventilation is crucial to control hypoxia resulting from a ventilatory disturbance. Managing a disruption in perfusion must concentrate on increasing blood flow through the pulmonary capillaries, the hemoglobin availability, and transport of oxygen to the cells.

Ventilation Regulation

Even though breathing can be changed voluntarily, ventilation is predominantly controlled involuntarily by the autonomic nervous system. A significant share of the rules linked to sustaining normal gas exchange and blood gas levels. The receptors within the body constantly measure the degree of oxygen (O_2), carbon dioxide (CO_2), and hydrogen ions (pH) that signal the brain to adjust the rate and depth of respiration (Figure 2-8). Centers responsible for ventilatory control are the:

- Chemoreceptors
- Lung receptors
- Specified centers in the brainstem

Chemoreceptors

Chemoreceptors are specific receptors that monitor the number of hydrogen ions (pH), carbon dioxide (CO_2) and oxygen (O_2) levels in the arterial blood. Chemoreceptors are two different types:

- **Central Chemoreceptors**
- **Peripheral Chemoreceptors**

Central Chemoreceptors

The central chemoreceptors positioned near the respiratory center in the medulla and are most sensitive to alterations of CO_2 (carbon dioxide) level in arterial blood as well as the pH of cerebrospinal fluid (CSF). It is essential to note that the pH of cerebrospinal fluid (CSF) directly linked to the volume of CO_2 (carbon dioxide) in the arterial blood. Carbon dioxide (CO_2) readily crosses the blood–brain barrier (BBB) and moves into the CSF. In the cerebrospinal fluid (CSF), the carbon dioxide (CO_2) combines with water (H_2O) to develop carbonic acid (H_2CO_3). Thus, there is a direct relationship between CO_2 and the acid level in the body as follows:

- An increase in the blood CO_2 increases the blood acid level.

- A decrease in the blood CO_2 decreases the blood acid level.

The central chemoreceptors are exceedingly sensitive to the hydrogen level in the CSF. After the combination of CO_2 and H_2O molecules to form H_2CO_3, the hydrogen ions (H^+) separate from the H_2CO_3, and enter the CSF, stimulating the central chemoreceptors. Small variations in the H^+ level in the CSF encourages a modification in respirations. Since CO_2 is needed to produce H_2CO_3, the alteration in the rate and depth of breathing are geared toward increasing or decreasing the level of CO_2 in the arterial blood. The ventilation reaction is briefed as follows:

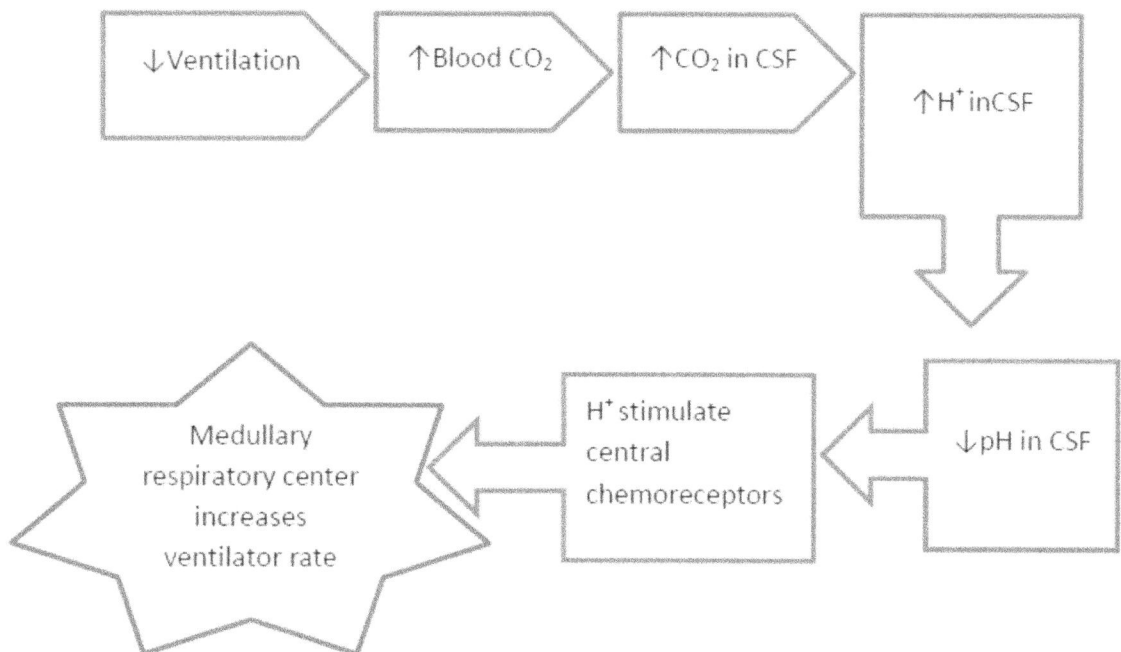

Figure 2-8 Mechanism of ventilation involving central chemoreceptors

- A rise in blood CO_2 ($PaCO_2$) increases the amount of hydrogen ions (H^+) in the cerebrospinal fluid (CSF), stimulating an increase in the rate and depth of respiration to exhale more CO_2.

- A reduction in $PaCO_2$ decreases the number of hydrogen ions (H^+) in the cerebrospinal fluid (CSF), causing a decrease in the rate, depth and pattern of respiration to exhale less CO_2.

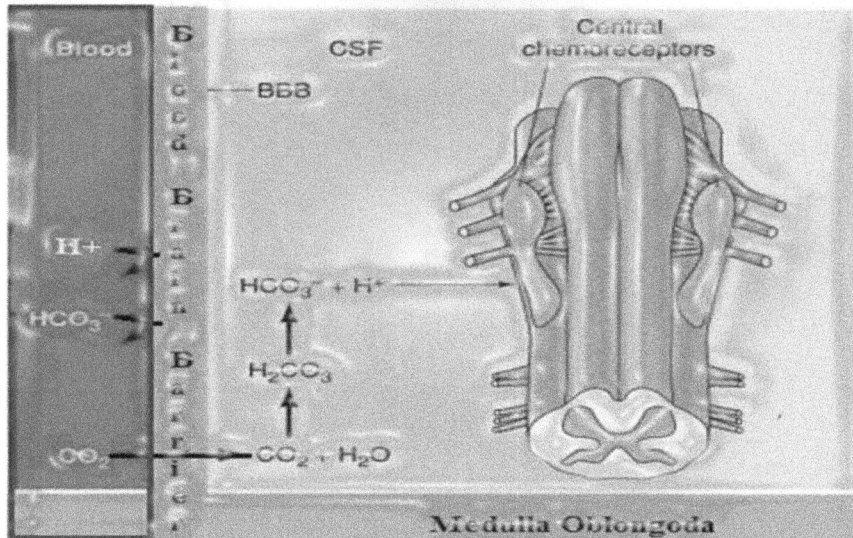

Figure 2-9   The association of the blood-brain barrier (BBB) to CO_2, HCO_3, and $H+$. CO_2 voluntarily crosses the BBB. $H+$ and HCO_3 do not freely cross the BBB. $H+$ and HCO_3 need the active transport system to cross the BBB. CSF = cerebrospinal fluid.

Peripheral Chemoreceptors

The peripheral chemoreceptors positioned in the carotid bodies in the neck and aortic arch. These chemoreceptors are also sensitive to CO_2 and the pH; however, the arterial oxygen level is the strongest stimulus. Thus, an alteration in the arterial oxygen level is what excites the brain to increase or decrease ventilation. It takes a substantial fall in the arterial oxygen content to elicit the peripheral chemoreceptors to excite the breathing center in the brain to increase the rate and the depth of breathing. Peripheral chemoreceptors activity can be summarized as follows:

- A substantial reduction in the arterial oxygen content causes an increase in the rate and depth of ventilation for the purpose of increasing the arterial oxygen content.

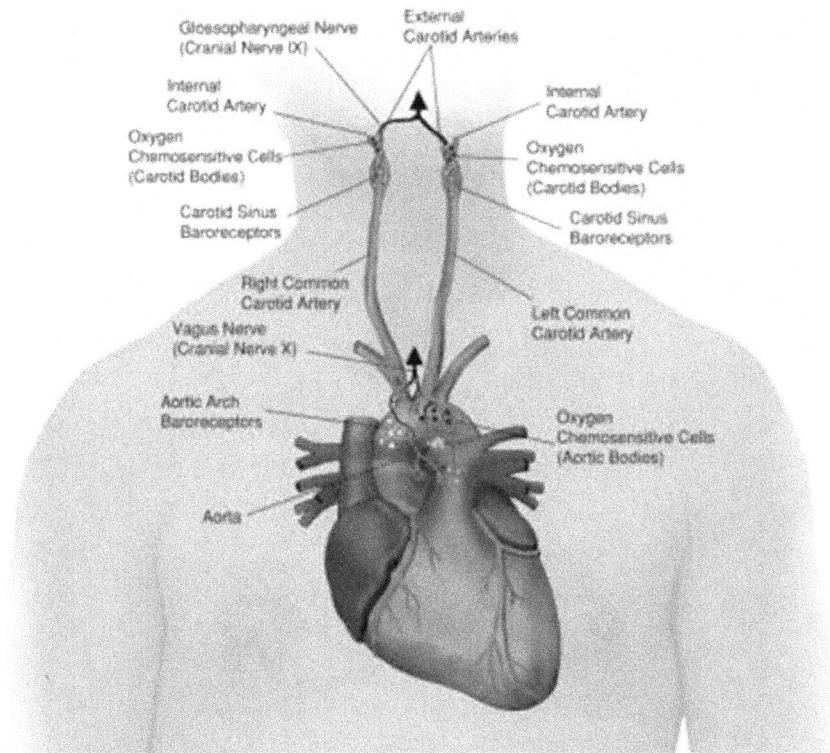

Figure 2-10   The site of the carotid and aortic bodies (the peripheral chemoreceptors). Source: Google images labeled for reuse by https://media.lanecc.edu/users/driscolln/RT127/Softchalk/regulation_of_Breathing/regulation_of_Breathing3.html

Altering the rate and depth of ventilation is significantly influenced by stimulation of both the central and peripheral chemoreceptors than one of them alone.

Receptors of the Lung

There are three different types of receptors or reflexes within the lungs:

- Irritant receptors,
- Stretch receptors or deflation reflex,
- Jaxtapulmonary-Capillary Receptors or J-receptors.

The **irritant receptors** found in the trachea, bronchi, and bronchioles. These receptors are sensitive to particles, noxious gasses, and aerosols that cause a cough, bronchoconstriction, and an increase in the rate of ventilation when exposed.

The **stretch receptors** or **deflation reflex** located within the smooth muscle of the airways. Stretch receptors are responsible for determining the size and capacity of the lungs. Furthermore, these receptors prevent overinflation in the case of high tidal volumes by decreasing the rate and volume of ventilation when stretched.

Juxtapulmonary-Capillary Receptors (J-receptors) located in the interstitial tissues between pulmonary capillaries surrounding the alveoli. These receptors are sensitive to increases in pressure within the capillary. When the J-receptors activated, the reflex responses by triggering shallow, rapid, breathing.

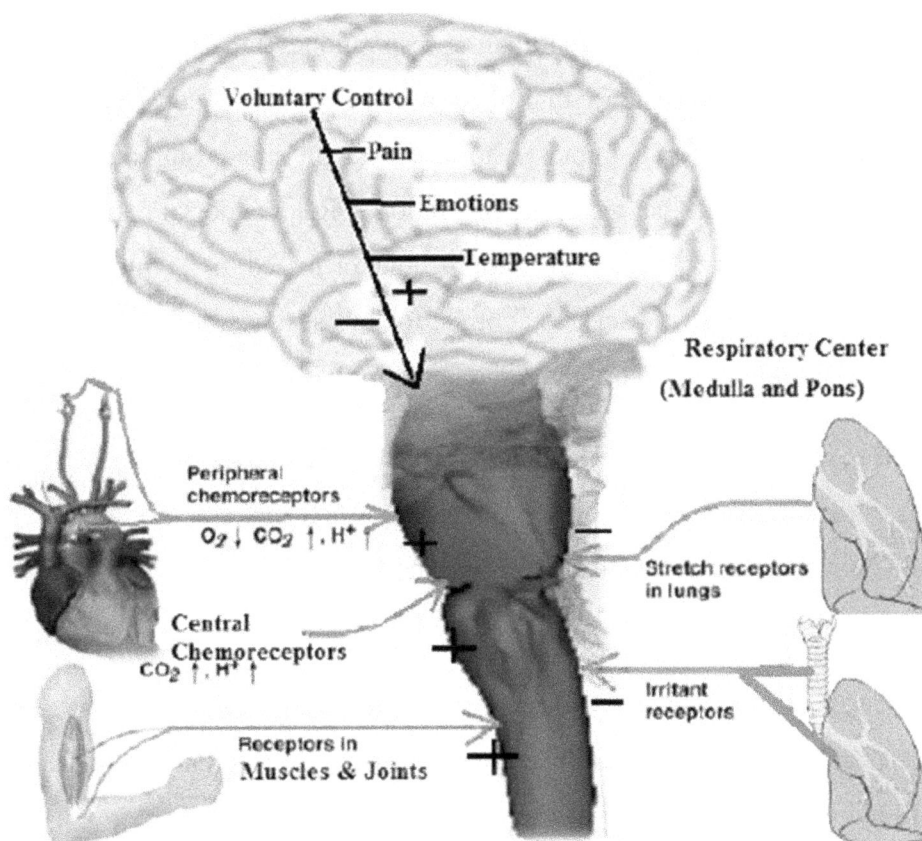

Figure 2-11 illustrates the receptors of the lungs, peripheral and central chemoreceptors and their function in the ventilation.

The brainstem contains four respiratory control centers:

- The dorsal respiratory group (DRG)
- The ventral respiratory group (VRG)
- The apneustic center (APC)
- The pneumotaxic Center (PNC)

These centers are responsible for coordinating respirations. (Fig. 2-12). The **dorsal respiratory group (DRG)** controls the basic rhythm of respiration. The DRG consists of inspiratory neurons responsible for sending nerve impulses to the external intercostal muscles and diaphragm, triggering them to contract, that results in inspiration. DRG, the dorsal respiratory group, is active in every respiratory phase, whether breathing is quiet or forced. In a typical respiratory cycle, the DRG excites the respiratory muscles to contract for two seconds, followed by three seconds with no stimulus, resulting in respiratory muscle relaxation.

The **ventral respiratory group (VRG)** has inspiratory and expiratory neurons. The VRG is non-functional during regular quiet breathing.However, when the accessory muscles are needed to assist in inspiration or expiration, the VRG becomes active.

The VRG_I, in which the subscript "I" specifies inspiratory VRG neurons, excites the pectoralis minor, scalene, and sternocleidomastoid muscles to force inspiration. The VRG_E, in which the "E" subscript specifies expiratory VRG neurons, triggers the internal intercostal and abdominal muscles to force exhalation.

The **apneustic center (APC)** does not control the respiration rhythm; however, it delivers stimulation to the DRG and VRG_I to increase the inhalation effort. The apneustic center may lengthen inspiration that leads to increasing ventilatory volume.

The **pneumotaxic Center (PNC)** directs inhibitory impulses to the apneustic center to terminate inhalation before the lungs become overinflated. It can stimulate passive exhalation both by shutting off the DRG and VRG_I and by triggering the VRG_E.

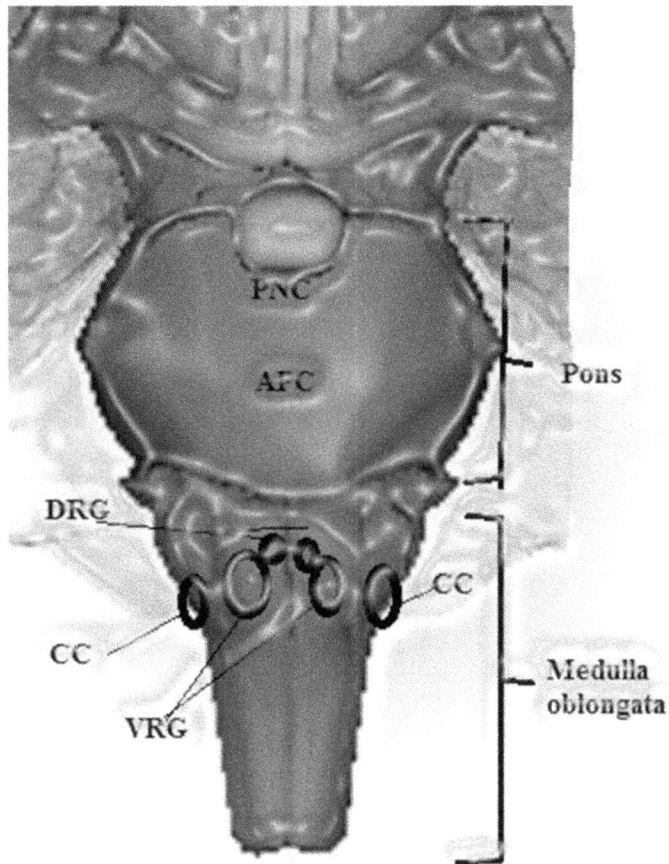

Figure 2-12: Graphic illustration of pons and medulla oblongata. PNC = pneumotaxic center; APC = apneustic center; DRG = dorsal respiratory group; VRG = ventral respiratory group; CC = central chemoreceptors.

Pulmonary Shunt

Pulmonary shunt classified into three types:

- Anatomic shunt (Fig. B)
- Capillary shunt (Fig. C)
- Shunt-like effect (Fig. D)

Anatomic shunt

Anatomic shunt occurs as the flow of blood from the right side of the heart transfers to the left side bypassing the alveolus for gas exchange. In the healthy lung, there is a normal anatomic shunt of about three percent of the cardiac output. Nonoxygenated blood produces the typical shunting of 3% entirely detouring the alveoli and entering (1) the pulmonary vascular system using the bronchial venous drainage and (2) the left atrium by way of the besian veins. Common abnormalities that cause anatomic shunting include congenital heart disease, intrapulmonary fistula, and vascular lung tumors. The figure below shows the normal alveolar-capillary unit(A) and anatomic shunt (B).

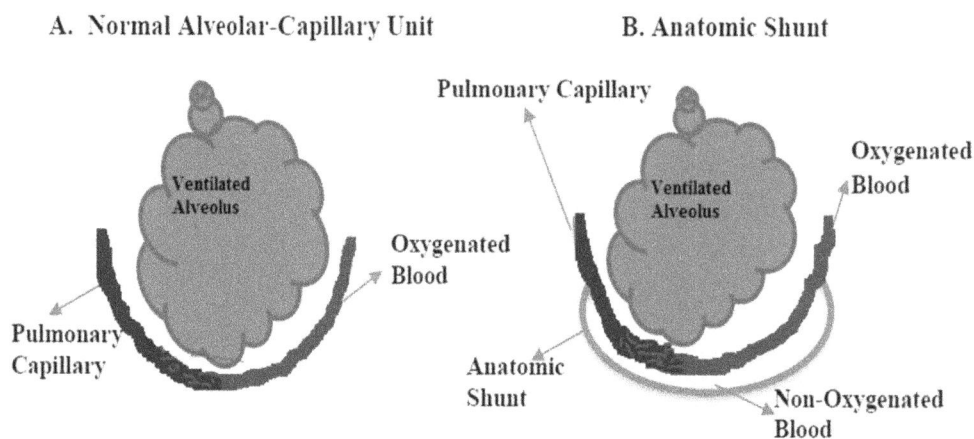

Figure 2-13: Displays A. Normal Alveolar-Capillary unit and B. Anatomic shunt

Capillary shunt

A capillary shunt is caused by alveolar collapse, atelectasis, alveolar fluid or consolidation. The combination of the anatomic and capillary shunt is known as a true or absolute shunt. Respiratory conditions causing capillary shunting circumstances will be refractory to oxygen therapy since the alveoli are unable to accommodate any form of ventilation as seen in figure 2-14.

C. Types of Capillary Shunts

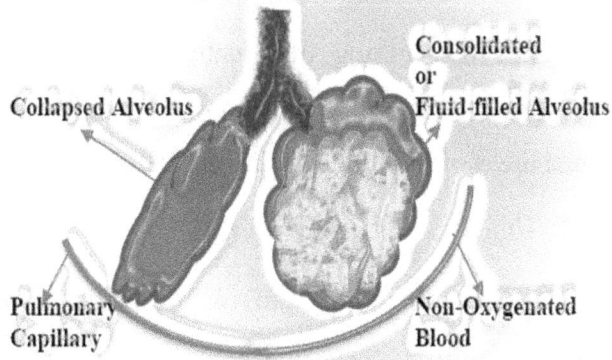

Figure 2-14 illustrates the Capillary shunts as the result of collapsed alveolus and consolidation.

Shunt-like effect or Relative shunt

Develops when pulmonary capillary perfusion is more than alveolar ventilation. This type of shunt commonly seen in patients with chronic obstructive lung disorders and alveolar-capillary diffusion defects. Also, called relative shunt, (Figure 2-15).

D. Types of Shunt-Like Effects

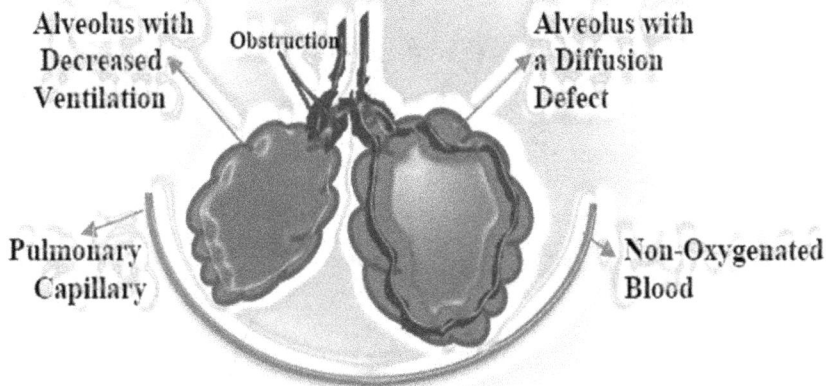

Figure 2-15: shows the shunt-like effects due to diffusion defect and obstruction.

Venous admixture   also called physiologic shunt or wasted blood flow

The venous admixture described as the mixing of shunted, non-reoxygenated blood with reoxygenated blood distal to the alveoli. Therefore, the blood flow entering the arterial system without passing through ventilated areas of the lung causing the PO_2 of arterial blood (PaO_2)to be less than that of alveolar PO_2 (PAO_2).

If shunt occurs, hypoxemia cannot be eliminated by providing the subject with 100% O_2. The arterial PO_2(PaO_2) is elevated slightly by an increase in dissolved O_2. A shunt, however, does not usually raise PCO_2 because chemoreceptors battle high PCO_2 with increased ventilation.

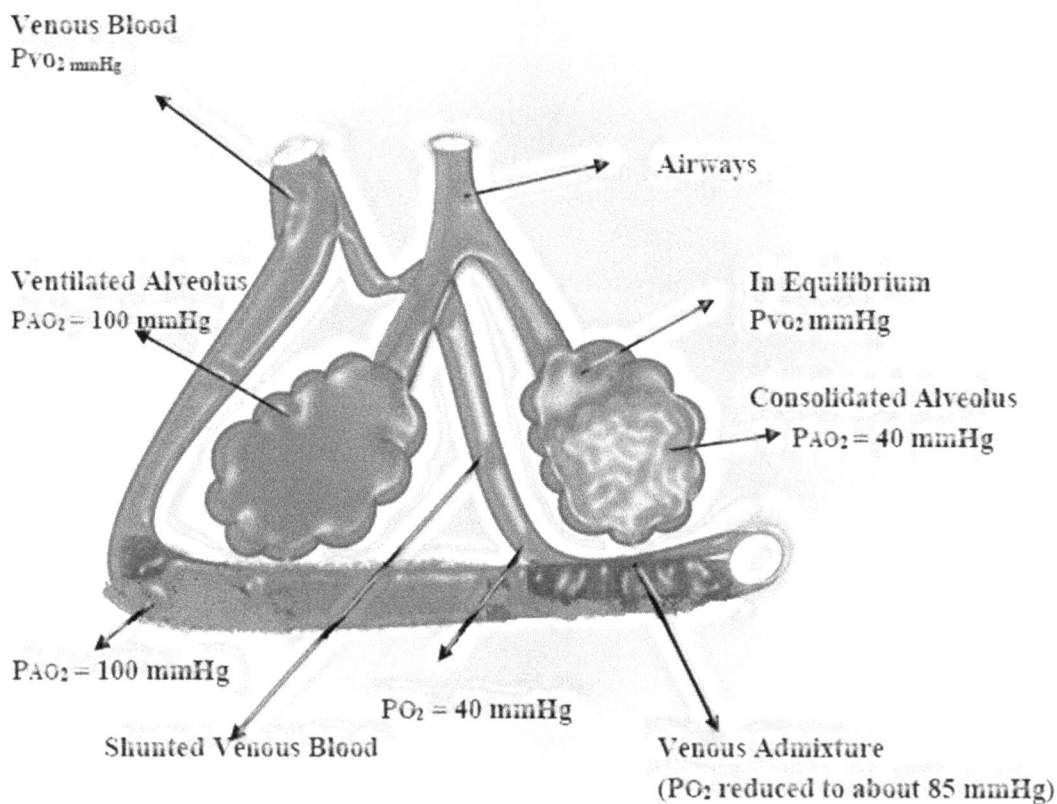

Figure 2-16: Displays venous admixture

TABLE 2-3: Classification of Respiratory Disorders associated with type of pulmonary shunt

Capillary Shunt	Stunt like effect	Combination Shunt
Pneumonia	Asthma	Cystic Fibrosis*
Pulmonary edema	Emphysema	Pneumoconiosis
ARDS	Chronic Bronchitis	Bronchiectasis*
Flail Chest	Croup and Epiglottitis	
Pneumothorax		
Pleural disease		
Kyphoscoliosis		
Tuberculosis		
Fungal Disease		
IRDS idiopathic respiratory distress syndrome		

Shunt Equation

It is evident that pulmonary shunt and venous admixture are common respiratory disorders; therefore, understanding the degree and amount of intrapulmonary shunt is valuable in developing patients care plan. The healthcare professionals can calculate shunt and obtain the necessary data through the standard shunt equation as seen in figure 2-17 below.

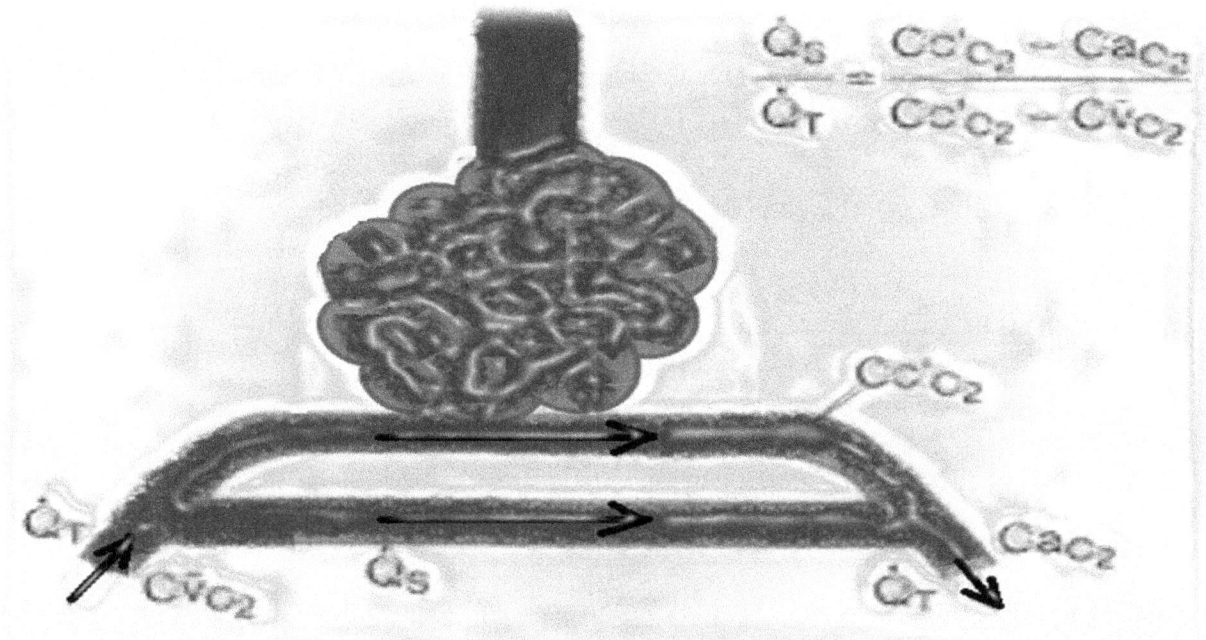

$$\frac{\dot{Q}_S}{\dot{Q}_T} = \frac{Cc'o_2 - Cao_2}{Cc'o_2 - C\bar{v}o_2}$$

Figure 2-17: illustrates the shunt equation

- Q_S is the Shunted cardiac output
- Q_T is the total cardiac output
- Oxygen content of arterial blood $\mathbf{Ca_{O2}}=(Hb \times 1.34 \times Sa_{O2}) + (Pa_{O2} \times .003)$
- Oxygen content of venous blood $\mathbf{Cv_{O2}}=(Hb \times 1.34 \times Sv_{O2}) + (Pv_{O2} \times .003)$
- Oxygen content of capillary blood $\mathbf{Cc_{O2}}=(Hb \times 1.34) + (P_{AO2} \times .003)$
- The partial pressure of alveolar oxygen $\mathbf{P_{AO2}}=[(PB-47) \times FiO_2] - (Pa_{CO2} \times 1.25)$

The following clinical information must be collected to calculate the shunt equation:

- **PB** Barometric pressure
- **Pa_{O2}** Partial Pressure of arterial oxygen
- **Pa_{CO2}** partial pressure of arterial carbon dioxide
- **Pv_{O2}** Partial pressure of mixed venous oxygen
- **Hb** Hemoglobin concentration
- **PA_{O2}** partial pressure of alveolar oxygen
- **FI_{O2}** Fractional concentration of inspired oxygen

Example:

Assumed the following information, calculate the % shunt: Hb 11 gm%, PB 750 torr, PaO_2 82 torr, SaO_2 94%, Pv_{O2} 36 torr, SvO_2 63%, $PaCO_2$ 40 torr, FiO_2 .40

- $\mathbf{Ca_{O2}} = (Hb \times 1.34 \times Sa_{O2}) + (PaO2 \times .003) = (11 \times 1.34 \times .94) + (82 \times .003) = 14.10$
- $\mathbf{Cv_{O2}} = (Hb \times 1.34 \times Sv_{O2}) + (PvO2 \times .003) = (11 \times 1.34 \times .63) + (36 \times .003) = 9.39$
- $\mathbf{PA_{O2}} = [(PB-47) \times Fi_{O2}] - (PaCO2 \times 1.25) = [(750-47) \times .4] - (40 \times 1.25) = 231.2$
- $\mathbf{Cc_{O2}} = (Hb \times 1.34) + (P_{AO2} \times .003) = (11 \times 1.34) + (231.2 \times .003) = 15.43$

$$\text{Shunt } (Qs/Q_T) = \frac{Cc_{O2} - Ca_{O2}}{Cc_{O2} - Cv_{O2}}$$

- **Shunt (Q_S/Q_T)** = (15.43-14.10) / (15.43-9.39) = 1.33/6.04 = 0.220 = 22.0%

Thus, 22.0% of the patient's pulmonary blood flow is perfusing lung tissue that is not being ventilated.

Clinical significance of pulmonary shunting is displayed in Table 2-4 below

Table 2-4 Clinical significance of pulmonary shunting

Degree of pulmonary shunt	Clinical implication
<10%	Normal Lung Status

10-20%	Pulmonary abnormality, but not significant regarding cardiopulmonary support
20-30%	Potentially life-threatening and cardiopulmonary support may be required
Greater than 30%	Serious life threatening situation and cardiopulmonary support are a must

Lung compliance

Compliance is a measure of the ease of expansion of the lungs and thorax, determined by pulmonary volume and elasticity. Lung compliance is measured regarding the change in unit volume (L) per unit pressure (cmH_2O) change. Therefore, Compliance determines the amount of air in liters the lung accommodates for each centimeter of water pressure change.

For example, during normal inspiration the negative intrapleural pressure change of 2 cmH_2O, the lung takes 0.2 liters of air that C_L is equal to 0.1 L/cmH_2O:

$$C_L \text{ (Compliance)} = \Delta V \text{ (L)} / \Delta P \text{ (cmH}_2\text{O)}$$
$$C_L = 0.2 \text{ L} / 2 \text{ cmH}_2\text{O}$$
$$C_L = 0.1 \text{ L/cmH}_2\text{O}$$

In a typical healthy lung at low volume, the comparatively little negative pressure outside (or positive pressure inside) needed to expand the lung. However, lung compliance declines with an increase in volume. Therefore, as the size of the lung increases, it requires applying more pressure to get the same increase in volume. This process is displayed on the following pressure-volume curve of the lung: Lung compliance and the slope are the same:

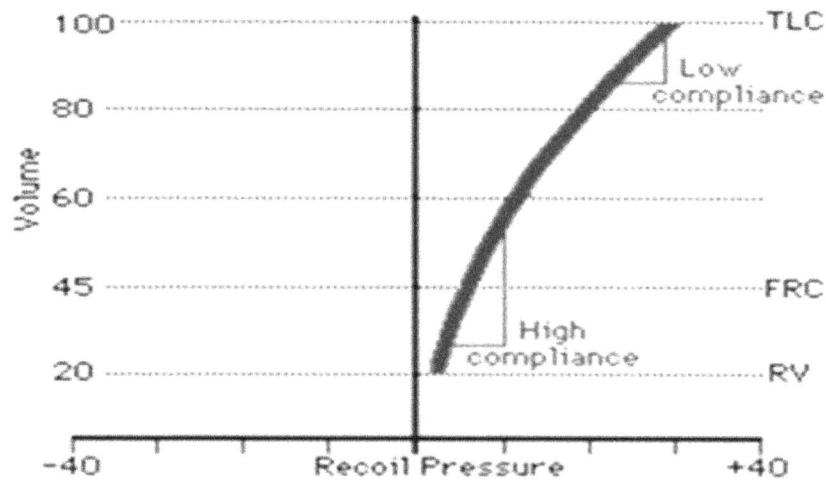

Figure 2-18: Pressure-Volume Curve of the lung: lung compliance and the slope showing low and high compliance. Source: http://oac.med.jhmi.edu/res_phys/Encyclopedia/Compliance/Compliance.HTML

A high grade of lung compliance specifies a loss of elastic recoil of the lungs, as in old age or emphysema. Thereby, lungs accept a greater volume of gas per unit of pressure.

Decreased lung compliance means that a greater change in pressure is needed for a given change in volume, as the lungs accept a smaller volume of gas per unit of pressure change such as in atelectasis, pneumonia, fibrosis, edema, or lack of surfactant. Dyspnea on exertion is the main symptom of reduced lung compliance.

Compliance can also alter in different disease conditions. For example, in fibrosis the lungs become rigid, making a tremendous pressure necessary to maintain a moderate volume, such lungs considered poorly compliant. On the other hand, in emphysema, due to the destruction of many alveolar walls, the lungs become very loose and floppy that only a slight pressure difference is required to retain a large volume. Thus, the emphysematous lungs considered highly compliant.

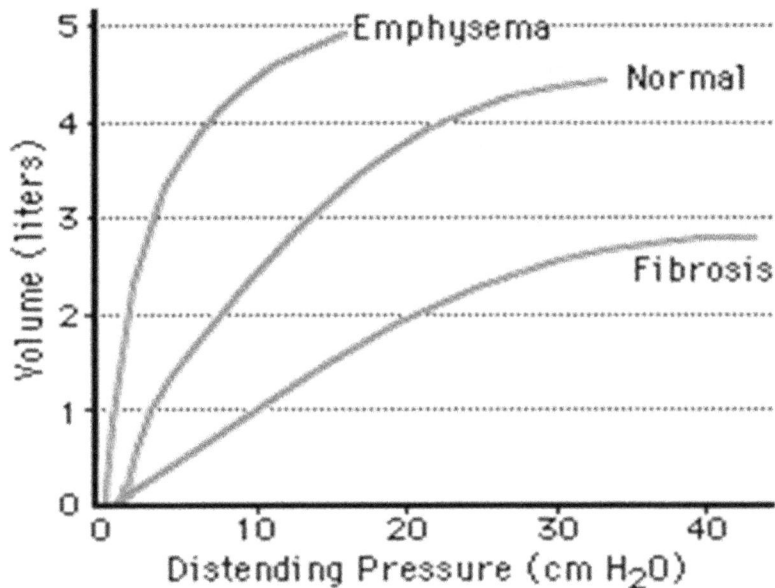

Figure 2-19: illustrates the effect of different diseases such as emphysema and fibrosis on the lung compliance. Source: http://oac.med.jhmi.edu/res_phys/Encyclopedia/Compliance/Compliance.HTML

Airway Resistance

Airway resistance is the difference of pressure between the mouth and the alveoli (trans airway pressure), divided by the flow rate. Airway resistance measured in centimeters of water per liter per second (cmH$_2$O/L/sec). The standard airway resistance in adults is about 0.5 to 1.5 cm H2O/L/sec. Higher airway resistance is seen in patients with chronic obstructive pulmonary disease (COPD) and infants.

The two ways air moves through the bronchial airways:

- Laminar flow is a smooth gas movement
  - ➢ the air molecules travel through the tubes in a form parallel to the sides of the bronchial tubes
  - ➢ It takes place at low flow rates and low-pressure gradients.
- Turbulent flow is a random gas current
  - ➢ The air encounters resistance from the tubes and other molecules.
  - ➢ It occurs at high flow rates and high-pressure gradients.

Laminar flow produced by Removal of obstructions and Correct flow rates

Turbulent flow caused by Obstructions, Excessive flow rates, Bifurcations

The impact of lung compliance and airway resistance on Ventilatory rate and pattern

Changes in lung compliance and airway resistance changes the ventilatory rate and pattern

Condition	Frequency (f)	Tidal Volume (V_T)
Decreased C_L	Increased	Decreased
Increased R_{aw}	Decreased	Increased

A Cough and Sputum Production

A cough is an abrupt, usually involuntary, expulsion of air from the lungs with a distinctive and easily detectable sound. While a cough is known as the most common symptom of respiratory conditions, it aids the functions of defending the respiratory tract against harmful substances and retaining airway patency by eliminating excessive secretions from the airway passages. Expectoration is sputum production which is the act of coughing up and spitting out the material produced in the respiratory tract.

Cough receptors are known as the rapidly adapting nerve endings, identified as irritant receptors. These nerve endings are more abundant in the mucosa of the larynx, carina, trachea, and large bronchi, that are readily stimulated by mechanical or chemical irritants. A cough is considered the most efficient form of airway secretion clearing method. Many other sites such as pharynx, peripheral airways, and intrathoracic or extrathoracic have demonstrated or suspected of cough receptors. For example, pleura, ear canals, tympanic membrane, and even the stomach comprise cough receptors. The vagus nerve is the most important afferent nerve, although the glossopharyngeal and trigeminal nerves may operate, depending on the receptors involved. A medullary cough center hypothesized with no evidence of its specific anatomic site. This "center" is under the effect of the higher voluntary nerve centers, which may initiate or change a cough. Vagi (recurrent laryngeals) are the efferent nerves, the phrenic nerves, and the spinal motor nerves of the expiratory muscles. Some factors that stimulate the irritant receptors are:

- Inflammation
- Mucus accumulation
- Noxious gasses such as cigarette smoke
- Chemical inhalation
- Very hot or cold air
- Mechanical stimulation such as endotracheal suctioning or compression of the airways.

The mechanical actions involved in a common cough are rapid progressions of:

- A fairly deep initial inspiration.
- The tight closure of the glottis that reinforced by the supraglottic structures.
- The quick and forceful contraction of the expiratory muscles.
- The immediate opening of the glottis while the contraction of the expiratory muscles continues.

The real high intrapulmonary pressure generated during the last two phases results in a very fast airflow from the lungs upon the opening of the glottis. Also, the difference between the outside pressure and the inside pressure of the intrathoracic airways during phase 4 causes their dynamic compression and narrowing. The high airflow combined with airway narrowing results in the expulsion of an airstream with a linear velocity is occasionally approaching the speed of sound. The explosion of air thus produced is capable of expelling the secretions with high force. The lung volumes determine the site and the extent of the dynamic compression. For example:

- Large lung volumes result in compression of only the trachea and large bronchi
- Small lung volumes cause more distal airways to narrow as well.

With each successive cough without an intervening inspiration, lung volumes become smaller, and the cough becomes effective in removing secretions from more distal airways, as seen in patients with chronic bronchitis. With the subsequent deep inspiration, the cough resumes with larger lung volumes, as the cough sequence recurse itself.

The explosive sound of a cough is due to:

- Vibrations of the vocal cords,
- Mucosal folds above and below the glottis,
- Accumulated secretions.

The numerous elements contributing to the distinction in cough sounds, including

- The nature and quantity of secretions.
- Anatomical variances and pathologic alteration of the larynx and other air passages.
- The force of a cough

Vibrations of coughing also assist in removing secretions from the airway walls.

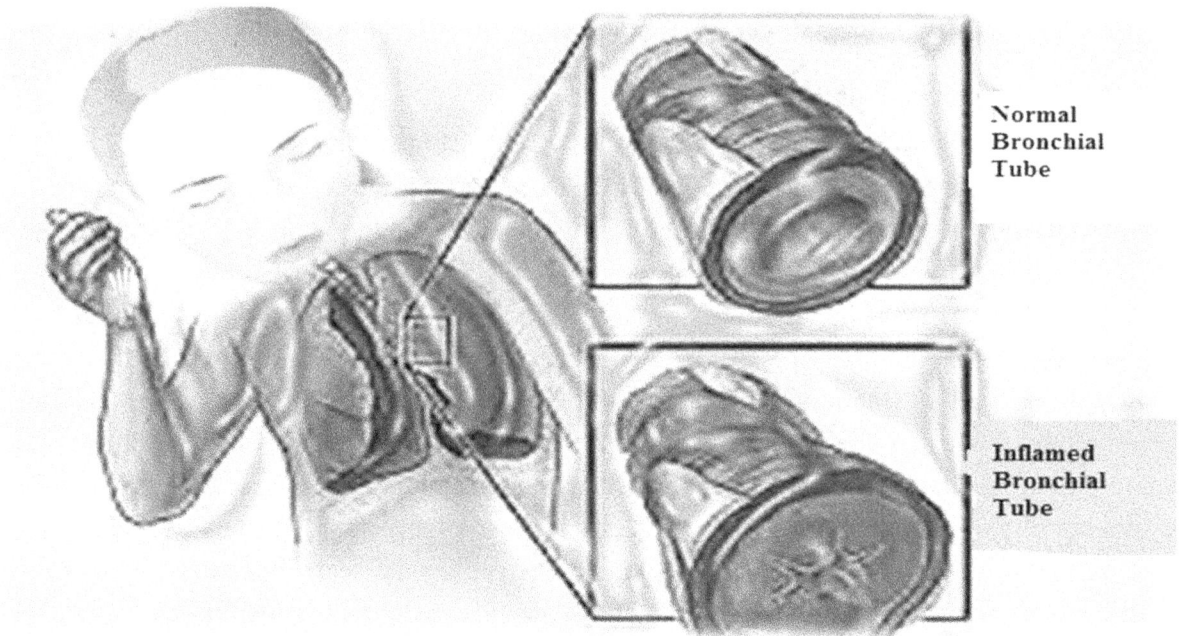

Figure 2-20 shows a cough and inflammatory response with mucus production.

Sputum Production

Respiratory mucus represents the products derived from the secretion of the tracheobronchial submucosal glands and the epithelial goblet cells,

whereas tracheobronchial secretions include the mucus plus other fluid and solute derived from the alveolar surface and the circulation. Sputum consists of bronchial mucus contaminated by saliva, transudated serum proteins, and inflammatory and desquamated epithelial cells. Sputum denotes an increase in normal secretions that is pathological.

The airways typically yield several ounces of sputum a day to keep breathing passageways moist. Once the lungs are bothered by irritants, extra mucus is produced to trap any inhaled particles from entering the lungs. Furthermore, Constant exposure to irritants, such as smoke, however, results in the enlargement of these glands and produce two to three times the usual volume of mucus. Chronic irritation impacts the natural cleaning system in the airways provided by the cilia. It is well known that smoking damages cilia. Smoking also causes any surviving cilia to become paralyzed for at least 20 minutes following inhalation of cigarette smoke. The result is a poorly working sweeping mechanism that doesn't clear the air passages very well.

The expectorated sputum may encompass other endogenous or exogenous materials in addition to mucus, including transudated or exudated fluids, necrotic tissues or cells, aspirated vomitus, various local or migrated cells, microorganisms, or additional foreign molecules.

The physical characteristics and gross appearance of the sputum are the results of its content of these and other materials. For example:

- Mucous sputum is clear in color or translucent and viscous, comprising only a small numbers of microscopic components.
- Purulent sputum is off-white, yellow, green, and perhaps cloudy and dense. It indicates the presence of a vast number of white blood cells, specifically neutrophilic granulocytes. For instance, in asthmatics, the eosinophilic cells causes sputum to look purulent.
- Red coloration, uniform or streaky, is typically the result of its mixture with blood.
- Carbon particles stain the sputum gray as in cigarette smokers or black as in coal miners or with smoke inhalation.

Characteristics of expectorated sputum frequently suggest the diagnosis of its cause. For example:

- Bronchiectasis is characterized by chronic expectoration of large amounts of purulent and foul-smelling sputum.
- Lung abscess specified as the abrupt production of indicated sputum in a febrile patient.
- Rusty colored purulent sputum indicates pneumococcal pneumonia.
- Klebsiella pneumonia characterized by currant jelly and sticky sputum.
- Blood-tinged frothy sputum displays pulmonary edema.

Hemoptysis:

Hemoptysis is expectorating blood or blood-tinged sputum from the respiratory tract. Hemoptysis occurs when small blood vessels that line the airways of the lungs are broken. The sputum is usually bright red and frothy with air bubbles. The repeated expectoration of blood-tinged sputum is associated with chronic bronchitis, bronchiectasis, cystic fibrosis, pulmonary embolism, infection, tuberculosis, fungal disease or more severe condition such as cancer of the lung. Massive Hemoptysis defined as coughing up 400-600 mL of blood within a 24-hour period.

Table 2-5 Summary of Causes of Hemoptysis

Bronchial disease	Parenchymal disease
<ul><li>Carcinoma</li><li>Bronchiectasis</li><li>Bronchitis</li><li>Bronchial edema</li><li>Foreign body</li></ul>	<ul><li>Tuberculosis</li><li>Pneumonia</li><li>Lung abscess</li><li>Fungal lung disease</li><li>Trauma</li><li>Actinomycosis</li><li>Mycetoma</li></ul>

Hemoptysis may be confused with Hematemesis, which is blood originates from the gastrointestinal tract and usually has a dark, coffee ground appearance.

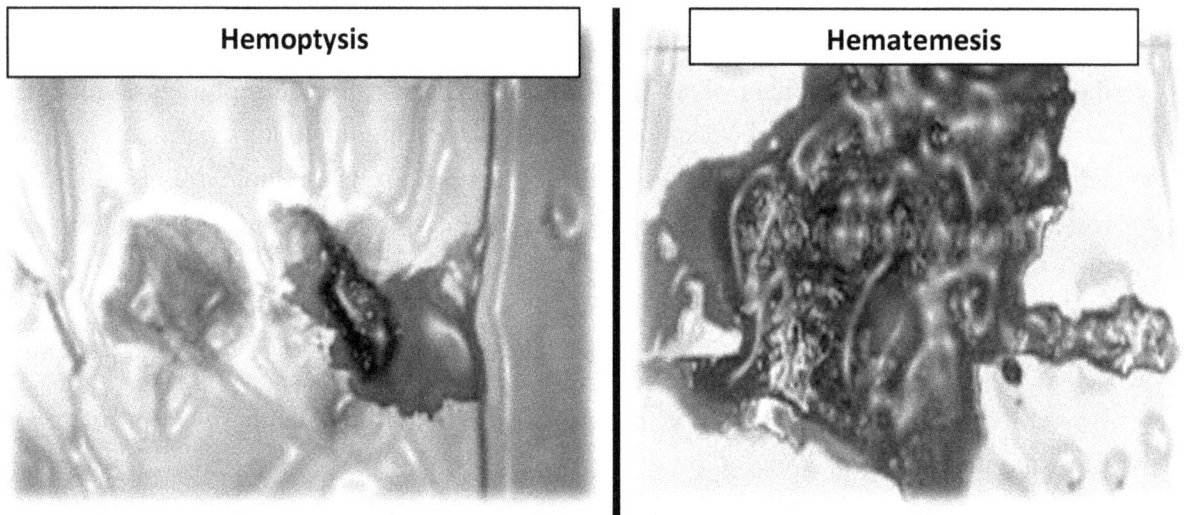

Figure 2-21 displays the difference in color and consistency of hemoptysis and hematemesis blood.

Table 2-6 Clinical Comparison of Hemoptysis and Hematemesis

Features	Hemoptysis	hematemesis
Sputum	**Color:** Bright red or Frothy pink **PH:** Alkaline **Consistency:** liquid with clotted appearance **Content:** Mixed with sputum	**Color:** Dark red or brown lower GI; Bright red upper GI usually not frothy **PH:** Acidic **Consistency:** Ground coffee, stale blood appearance **Content:** may have food particles
History	No nausea and vomiting may have history of lung disease Possibly associated with coughing or gurgling	Presence of nausea and vomiting Possible history of GI or Hepatic disease

Barrel Chest or Increased Anteroposterior Chest Diameter

Barrel chest results from a long-term overinflation of the lungs causing a rounded, bulging, almost barrel-like appearance of the chest. Furthermore, the lungs are overinflated with air causing the rib cage to stay partially expanded, giving the distinctive appearance of a barrel chest. Therefore, this condition results in an increased anteroposterior chest diameter.

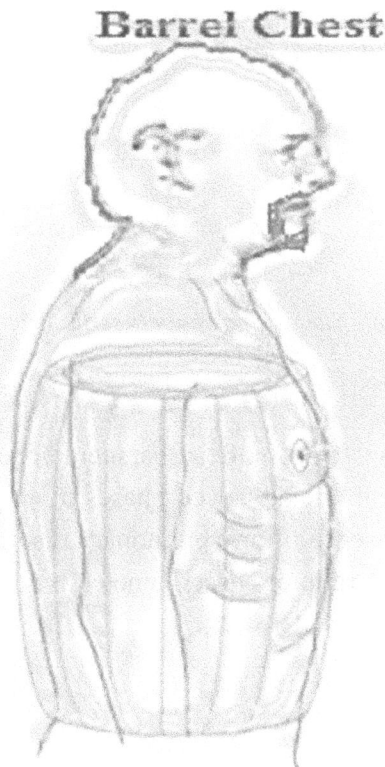

Figure 2-22: shows the appearance of barrel chest with increased anteroposterior chest diameter

Usually, the anteroposterior diameter of the chest is about half the lateral diameter as 1:2 ratios. In barrel chest, the ratio becomes almost 1:1 ratio.

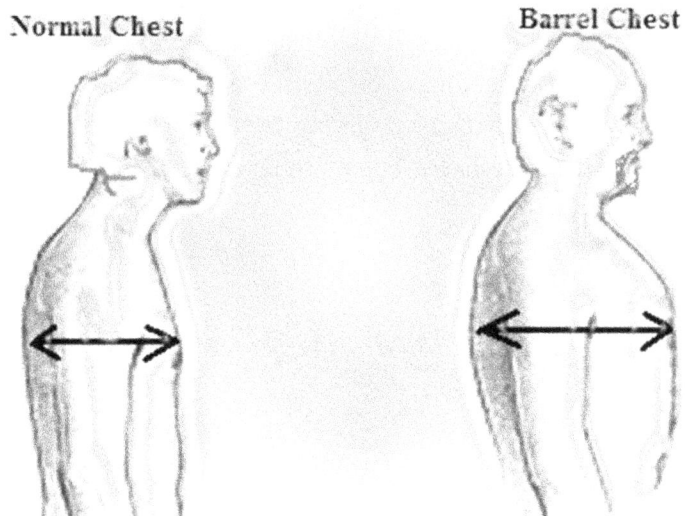

Figure 2-23: shows the comparison of normal chest diameter and Barrel chest diameter

Barrel chest can be the result of a variation of causes, including aging and osteoarthritis; however, barrel chest is a common finding in the advanced phases of emphysema. Thus, older individuals may have a barrel chest in the absence of any pulmonary disorders. It is notable that the normal newborn infants usually have a 1:1 ratio of chest diameter as well.

Pursed-Lip Breathing (PLB)

One of the easiest ways to control shortness of breath is through pursed-lip breathing. PLB provides a rapid and easy way to slow the pace of respiration, making each breath more efficient.

Pursed-Lip Breathing (PLB) creates back-pressure inside the airways to keep them open to ease the movement of air with less effort.

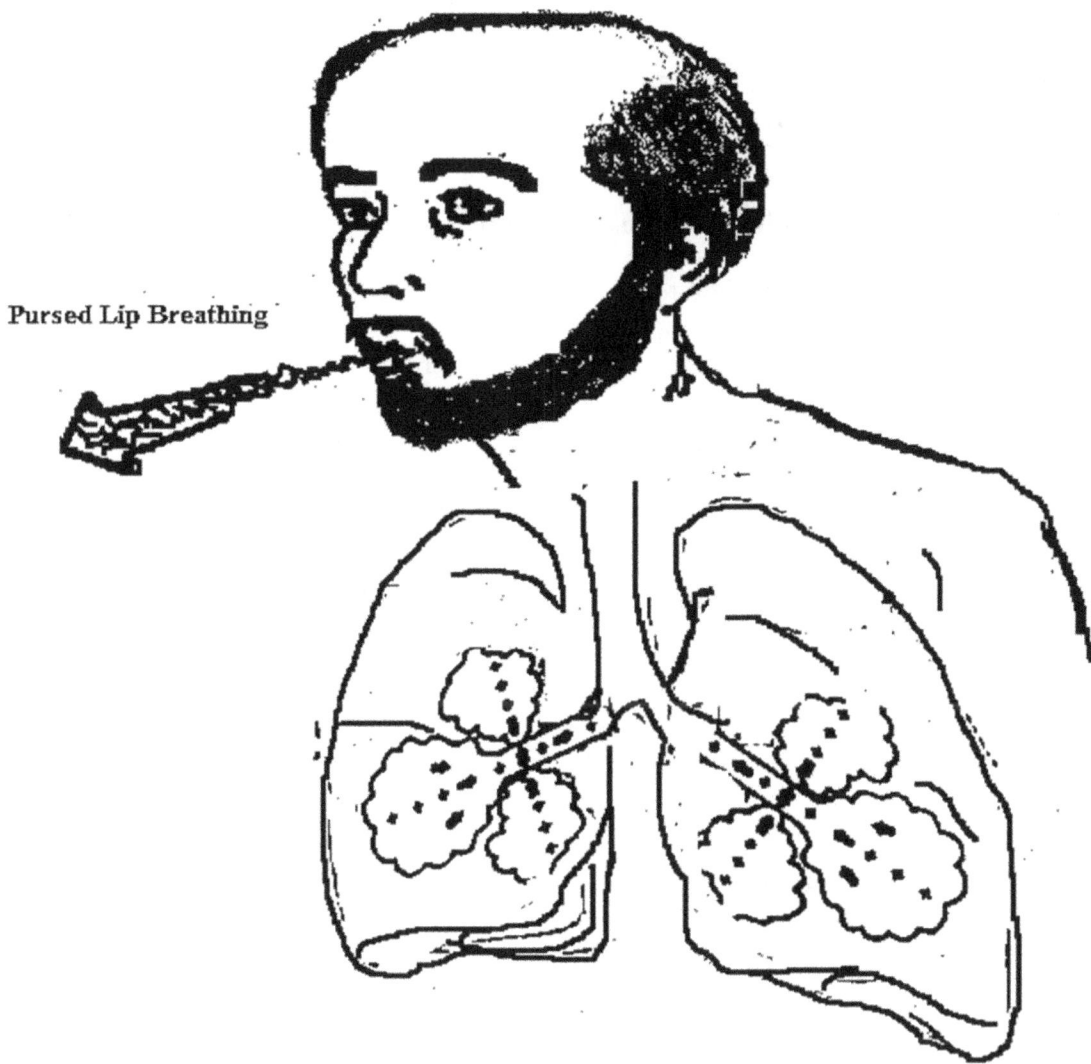

Pursed Lip Breathing

Figure 2-24: shows the pursed lip breathing in creating back-pressure in the airways and lungs to keep them open for the ease of air movement

A significant tenacity of PLB is to improve exhalation. PLB relieves some strain on over-stretched chest muscles and some work of breathing and returns the inhalation-to-exhalation ratio toward a normal 1:2. Thus, pursed lip breathing increases the efficiency of air exchange and enhances exercise tolerance. Some of the benefits of pursed lip breathing are:

- Improves patients' ventilation
- Releases trapped air in the lungs
- Maintains clear airways longer and reduces the work of breathing
- Protracts exhalation to slow the breathing rate

- Eases breathing patterns by moving old or trapped air out of the lungs and permitting for new air to enter the lungs
- Relieves shortness of breath
- Causes general relaxation

Steps in performing pursed lip breathing technique:

1. The patient should inhale slowly through the nose for two counts.

2. The patient should feel the abdomen distends during inhalation.

3. Pucker the lips as to whistle or blow out a candle.

4. The patient should exhale slowly through the puckered lips for 4 or more counts.

Exhalation should be normal without forcing the air out. The patient should not hold breath during pursed lip breathing. The steps should be Repeat until the breathing slows. These steps are shown in figure 2-25, Below.

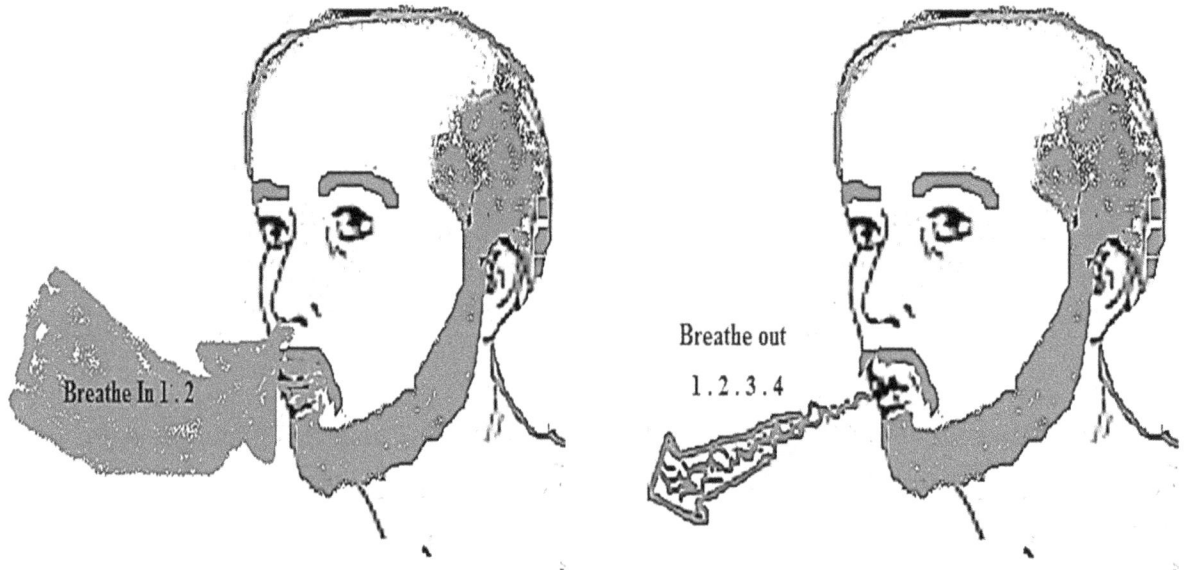

Figure 2-25: Pursed-lip breathing technique

Polycythemia, Cor-Pulmonale

Polycythemia is an increased level of red blood cells RBC. Pulmonary disorders produce chronic hypoxemia thereby the hormone erythropoietin responds by stimulating the bone marrow to increase the red blood cell, RBC, production as called erythropoiesis. The polycythemia caused by hypoxemia is an adaptive mechanism that increases the oxygen-carrying capacity of the blood.

Cor-Pulmonale is the alteration of right ventricular structure or function that is due to pulmonary hypertension as the result of diseases affecting the lung or its vasculature. Cor-Pulmonale defined as right ventricular hypertrophy that increases right ventricular work and leads to right ventricular failure.

The two major mechanisms involved in producing Cor-Pulmonale in chronic pulmonary disease are:

- Polycythemia causes increased viscosity of the blood.

- Hypoxic Vasoconstriction causing increase pulmonary vascular resistance.

Leading causes of Cor-Pulmonale are:

Lung disease

> Chronic obstructive pulmonary disease
> Cystic fibrosis
> Interstitial lung diseases

Disorders of the pulmonary circulation

> Pulmonary thromboembolism
> Primary pulmonary hypertension
> Tumor emboli
> Sickle cell anemia
> Schistosomiasis
> Pulmonary veno-occlusive disease

Neuromuscular diseases

> Amyotrophic lateral sclerosis
> Myasthenia gravis
> Poliomyelitis
> Guillain-Barre syndrome
> Spinal cord lesions
> Bilateral diaphragmatic paralysis

Thoracic cage deformities

Kyphoscoliosis

Disorders of Ventilatory control

Primary central hypoventilation
Sleep apnea syndromes

Pathophysiology of Cor-Pulmonale

Alveolar Hypoxia and Vasoconstriction of Pulmonary Vascular System

Chronic respiratory disorders cause a decrease in arterial oxygen level thereby results in contraction of the smooth muscle of the pulmonary arterioles. Hypoxemia and academia resulting from pulmonary disease creates generalized pulmonary vasoconstriction in which leads to increase vascular resistance and pulmonary hypertrophy causing increased right ventricular afterload. This process, in turn, can lead to right ventricular hypertrophy and Cor-Pulmonale.

Polycythemia and Increase Blood Viscosity

The advantage of Polycythemia in increasing oxygen carrying capacity is offset by the increased viscosity of the blood when hematocrit reaches about 50-60 percent. Increased viscosity of the blood requires greater driving pressure to maintain blood flow. Consequently, the right ventricle must work harder to produce the needed pressure to overcome the increased viscosity leading to pulmonary hypertension and increase right ventricular afterload. This rise in demand on right ventricle leads to right ventricular hypertrophy, called Cor-Pulmonale.

Consequently, the Cor-Pulmonale occurs as a result of hypoxemia associated with the chronic respiratory disorder may develop from the combined effect of polycythemia and pulmonary vasoconstriction. In Cor-Pulmonale as the right heart weakens causing the venous blood to accumulate in the large vessels as manifested by distended neck veins, enlarged and tender liver, and edema in the lower extremities.

The summary of Pathophysiology of Cor-Pulmonale is displayed in figure 2-26 below:

Pathophysiology of Cor pulmonale

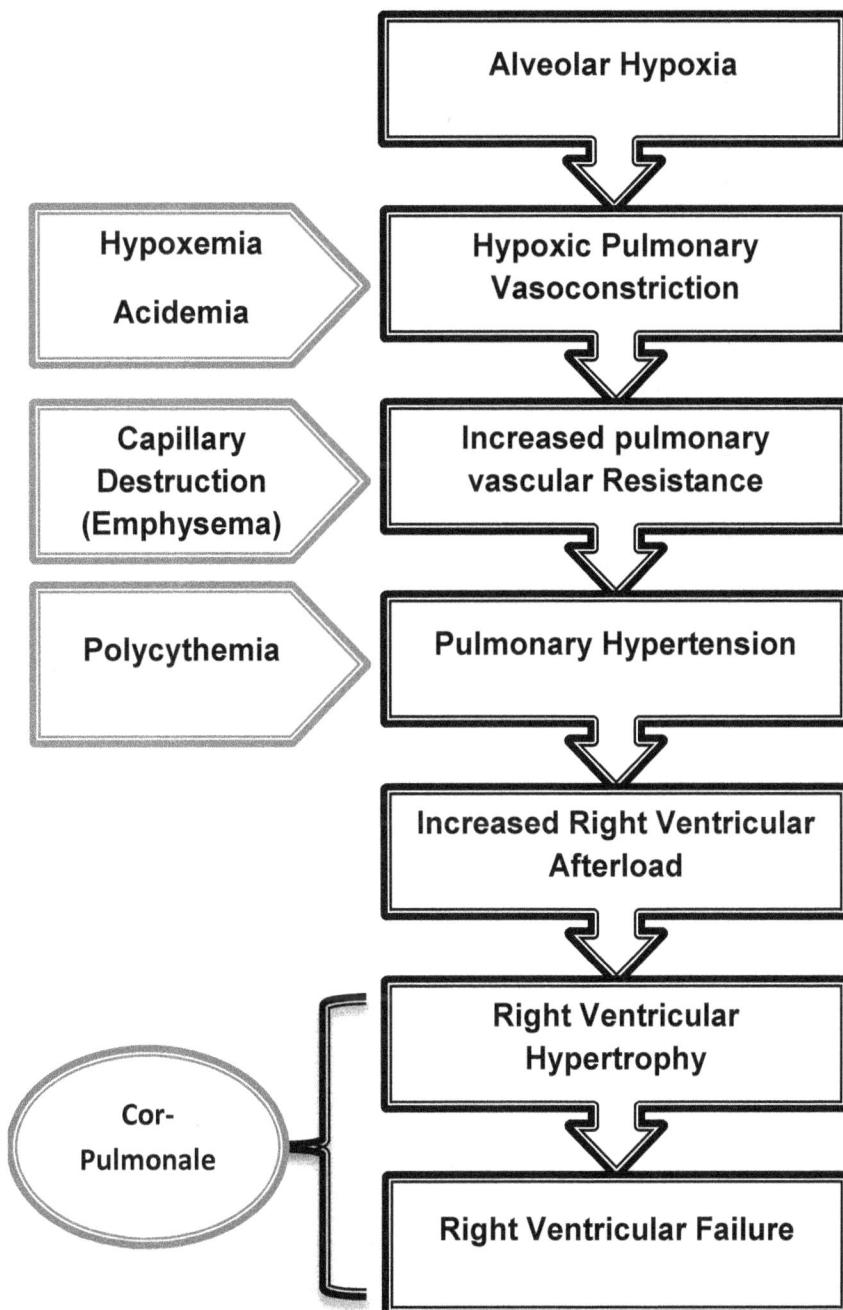

Figure 2-26: illustrates the pathophysiology of Cor-Pulmonale

Digital Clubbing

Digital clubbing is described by a focal bulbous enlargement of the terminal segments of the fingers and/or toes due to the proliferation of connective tissue between nail matrix and the distal phalanx. It results in an increase in both anteroposterior and lateral diameter of the nails. Clubbed fingers are also known as watch-glass nails, drumstick fingers, and Hippocratic fingers/nails.

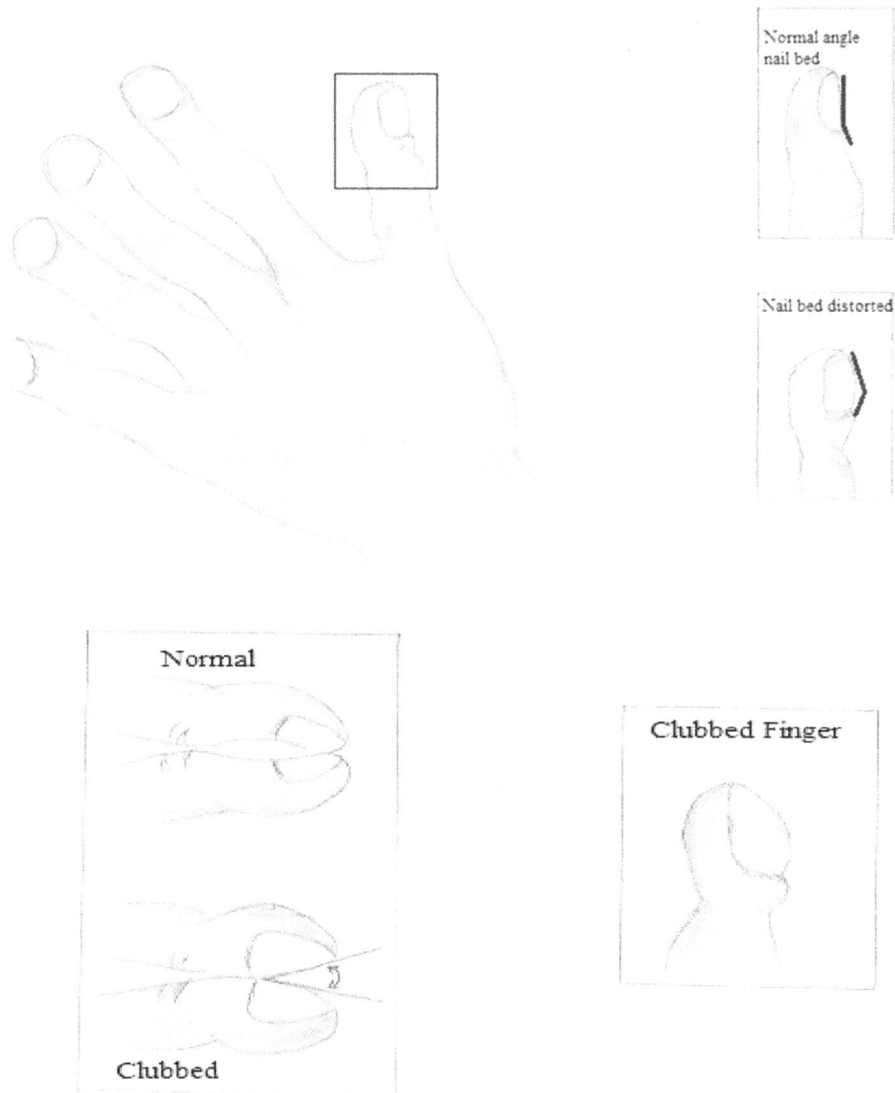

Figure 2-27: Displays the digital clubbing of finger and the comparison to the normal angle of nail bed

Digital clubbing associated with a variety of clinical conditions. However, lung diseases are most commonly associated with clubbing. Subsequently, neoplastic lung disease is the most common pulmonary cause of clubbing.

The exact pathophysiological mechanism for each cause of clubbing is unknown. However, the following factors are identified as a possible cause:

- Arterial and local hypoxia
- Circulating vasodilators such as bradykinin and prostaglandins, that are released from normal tissues.
- Chronic infection
- Capillary stasis from increased venous back pressure
- Unspecific toxins

Treatment of underlying disease may result in resolution of clubbing and return of the digits to normal.

Arterial Blood Gasses

An arterial blood sample is used for an arterial blood gas (ABG) test; arterial blood contains the oxygen and carbon dioxide levels that can be measured before they enter body tissues.

An ABG test measures:

- **The partial pressure of oxygen (PaO$_2$).** The PaO$_2$ measures the pressure of oxygen dissolved in the blood and displays the proficiency in diffusing of oxygen from the airspace of the lungs into the blood stream.
- **The partial pressure of carbon dioxide (PaCO$_2$).** The PaCO$_2$ measures the pressure of carbon dioxide dissolved in the blood and shows the effectiveness of leaving carbon dioxide from the body.
- **The pH** level indicates the hydrogen ions (H+) in blood. The pH of blood is typically between 7.35 and 7.45. When a pH level goes below 7.0 is called acidic, and a pH greater than 7.0 is called basic (alkaline). Thus blood is marginally basic.
- **The Bicarbonate (HCO$_3$)** is a chemical (buffer) that neutralizes the pH of the blood from becoming too acidic or too basic.
- **The Oxygen content (O$_2$CT)** and **oxygen saturation (SO$_2$) values.**
  - ➢ O2 content measures the amount of oxygen in the blood.
  - ➢ Oxygen saturation measures the percentage of the hemoglobin binding sites in the red blood cells is occupied by oxygen (O$_2$).

The ABG measurement is a vital information when caring for patients with critical illness or respiratory disease.

Arterial Sampling and Puncture Sites

The criteria for choosing the best puncture site are collateral blood flow and vessel accessibility as there are three primary sites for obtaining an arterial blood gas:

Radial Site: Blood is usually withdrawn from the radial artery as it is easy to palpate and has a good collateral supply. The radial site is the first choice as it meets the above criteria the best.

Brachial Site: which is the inside of the arm above the elbow crease and it is called brachial artery. The brachial site is an appropriate alternative site or the second choice.

Femoral Site: Blood can also be taken from an artery in the groin called femoral artery.

Before the procedure a test called the **Allen test** may be conducted to ensure collateral blood flow to the hand is normal. The steps in performing **Allen's test** are as follows:

- Instruct the patient to tighten his/her fist, or if the patient is unable, the practitioner may close patient's hand tightly.
- Using two fingers (thumbs), apply occlusive pressure to both the ulnar and radial arteries. This operation impedes blood flow to the hand.
- At the same time as the occlusive pressure applied to both the arteries, the patient is asked to relax his/her hand. The palm and fingers should become pale. (If it does not, practitioner have not completely occluded the arteries with his/her fingers).
- Release the occlusive pressure on the ulnar artery. The practitioner should notice a flushing of the hand within 5 to 15 seconds. The blushing of hand signifies that the ulnar artery is patent and has good blood flow. This natural blushing of the hand is considered to be a positive modified Allen's test.
- A negative modified Allen's test is one in which the hand does not flush within the specified period. This situation indicates that ulnar circulation is inadequate or nonexistence. The radial artery supplying arterial blood to that hand should not be punctured.

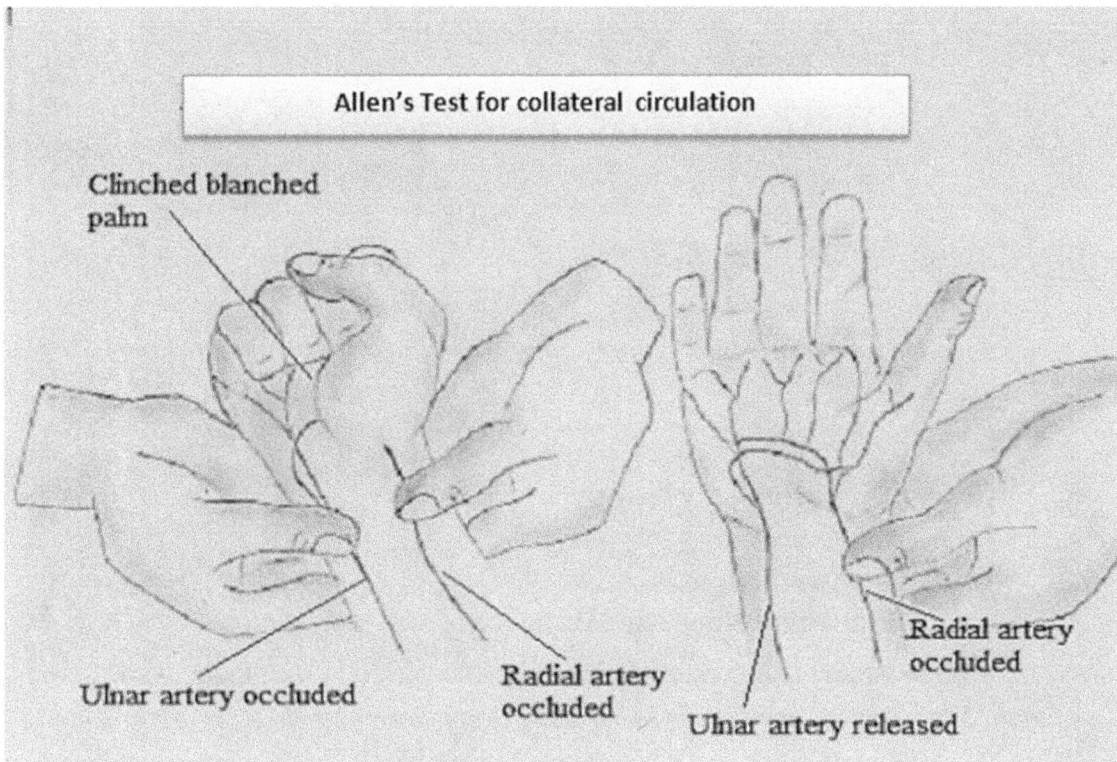

Figure 2-28: Displays Allen's test for collateral circulation

An arterial blood gas (ABG) test must not be performed on a site or an arm used for dialysis; Similarly, if there is an infection or inflammation in the area of the puncture site.

Steps in obtaining arterial blood gas:

- The patient's arm is positioned palm-up on a flat surface, with the wrist dorsiflexed at 45°.
- A small towel may be placed under the wrist for support.
- The puncture site must be cleaned with alcohol or iodine.
- Palpate The radial artery for a pulse, and a pre-heparinized syringe with a 23 or 25-gauge needle is inserted at an angle just distal to the palpated pulse.
- A small quantity of blood is sufficient usually about 1-2cc.
- After the puncture, to obtain haemostasis, direct pressure should be applied firmly by placing a sterile gauze over the puncture site for several minutes.

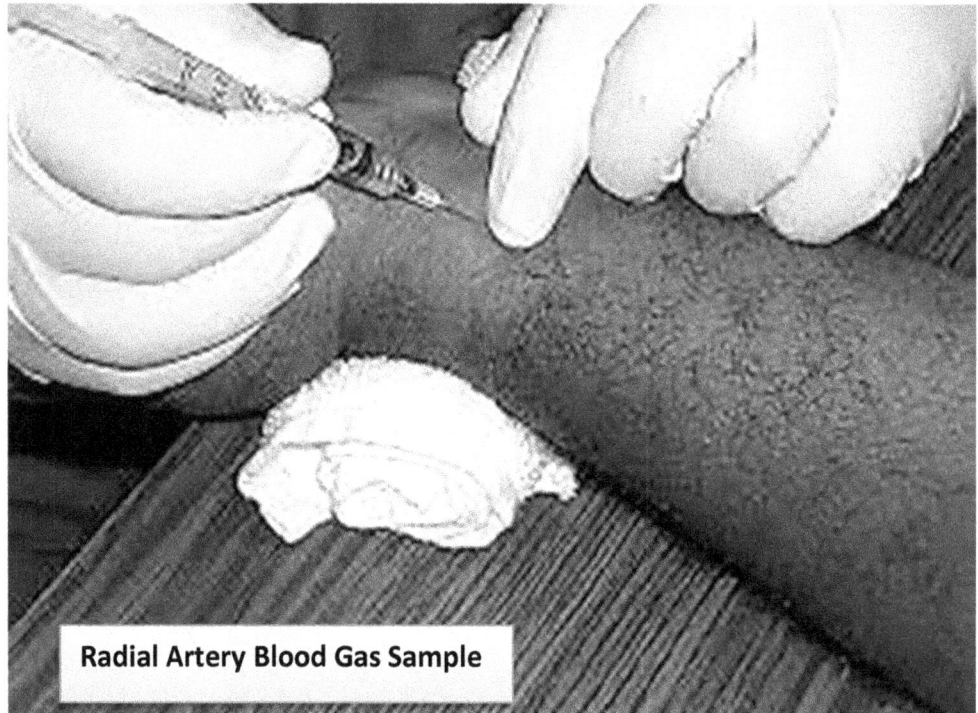

Figure 2-29: shows the puncture of radial artery to obtain arterial blood for (ABG) analysis. Source: http://slideplayer.com/slide/2497881/

When a repeated arterial blood gas needed, it is prudent to use a different site such as the other artery or perhaps insert an arterial line to prevent trauma to the site.

It is essential to analyze the sample promptly to ensure the accuracy of the ABG results. For any delay in processing the sample, the blood must be stored on ice at zero degrees for approximately 30 minutes. Hence, the ice and low temperature preserve the blood and the accuracy of the results for the indicated time limit.

Even though the complications from an arterial puncture are rare; they can include prolonged bleeding, infection, thrombosis or arteriospasm.

Normal arterial blood gas value is displayed in the table below:

Table 2-7: Normal blood gas value

Normal ABG Values

Analyte	Normal Value	Normal Range*
pH	7.40	7.35 to 7.45
$PaCO_2$ (mmHg)	40	35 to 45
HCO_3^- (mmol/L)	24	21 to 28
PaO_2 (mmHg)	100	80 to 110

Normal room air ABGs can be evaluated by adding the PO_2 and PCO_2 the total should be between 110 and 140.

- Values lower than 110 may indicate V/Q mismatch, diffusion defect, shunting or venous blood.
- Values higher than 140 would indicate supplemental oxygen in use, an air bubble in the sample, or technical error.

Factors affecting the ABG values:

- Temperature Corrections: blood gasses are typically reported as the standard body temperature of 37 degrees Celsius. Therefore, if the patient has an abnormal temperature, correction should be made. For example, if body temperature is high such as fever and machine analyzer is not corrected then the result will be altered as follow:
  - High temp = Lower CO_2, Lower PO_2, and Higher pH than the corrected results
  - Lower temp as Hypothermic = Higher CO_2, Higher PO_2, and Lower pH than the corrected results

- Air bubble in sample results in:
  - Increase or decrease PO_2
  - Decrease PCO_2
  - Increase pH

- Improper cooling:
  - Decrease PO_2
  - Increase PCO_2
  - Decrease pH

- Excessive Heparin:
  - Decrease pH
  - Decrease PCO_2
  - Increase PO_2

Table 2-8: Factors affecting ABG Values

Factors	pH	PCO_2	PO_2
Temperature			
High Temp	↑	↓	↓
Low Temp	↓	↑	↑
Air Bubble	↑	↓	↓↑
Improper Cooling	↓	↑	↓
Excessive Heparin	↓	↓	↑

The three most critical approaches to the interpretation of arterial blood gas (ABG) are as follows:

- Ventilation- $PaCO_2$
- Oxygenation- PaO_2, FIO_2
- Acid-Base Balance- PH
  - Acidosis VS Alkalosis
  - Compensated VS Uncompensated
  - Respiratory VS Metabolic

Ventilation, as indicated by PaCO2, is breathing air into and out of the lungs. The normal $PaCO_2$ is 35-45 mmHg (torr) signifying normal ventilation. As the $PaCO_2$ increase above 45 mmHg or torr ventilation becomes inadequate indicating hypoventilation requiring a response to increasing ventilation. However, when the $PaCO_2$ decrease below 35mmHg, it indicates hyperventilation. See table 2-9 below.

Table 2-9: Ventilation-$PaCO_2$ status

ABG- $PaCO_2$ Value	Indication	Response
35-45 torr	Normal Ventilation	Check Oxygen
Above 45 torr	Hypoventilation (Patient not ventilating)	Ventilate patient or increase ventilation
Below 35 torr	Hyperventilation (patient is ventilating too much)	Check oxygen

Oxygenation – PaO_2, FIO_2

The normal PaO2 is 80-100torr on FIO_2 of 0.21-0.59 and considered as an acceptable oxygenation. ABG value of below 80torr at FIO_2 of 0.21-0.59 suggests hypoxemia due to poor ventilation (high PCO_2) and V/Q mismatch (normal PCO_2) in these cases both increase ventilation and increase FiO2 is required. Also, PaO2 of below 80 torr at FIO2 higher than 0.60 indicates shunt; shunt, in this instance, requires higher PEEP or CPAP therapy.

ABG value of PaO_2 above 100 torr at FIO_2 of 0.22-1.0 is suggestive of over oxygenation the response to this situation would be to decrease FIO_2, PEEP or CPAP. Simplification of oxygenation is displayed in table 2-10 below

Table 2-10: Oxygentation-PaO2, FIO$_2$ values and their indications

ABG- PaO$_2$ Value	FIO$_2$	Indication	Response
80-100 torr	.21-.59	Acceptable Oxygenation	Maintain settings
Below 80 torr	.21-.59	Hypoxemia: poor ventilation (high PCO2)	Increase ventilation
		V/Q mismatch (normal PCO2)	Increase FIO$_2$
Below 80 torr	0.60 or higher	Shunting	Start or increase PEEP/CPAP therapy
Above 100 torr	.22-1.0	Over oxygenation	Decrease FIO$_2$, PEEP, CPAP

Decrease the FIO$_2$ first if .60 or above, then reduce the CPAP or PEEP

Acid-Base Balance- pH

To function properly Blood needs the right balance of acid and basic (alkaline) composites which refers to as the acid-base balance. The acid-base balance is the effort of the lungs, and the kidneys working together. Even slight variations from the normal range can have significant effects on the body's essential organs.

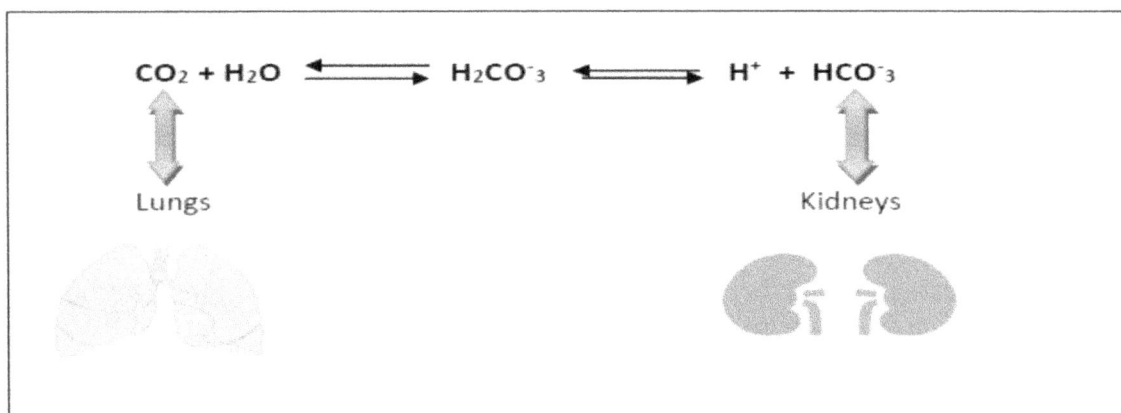

$$CO_2 + H_2O \rightleftharpoons H_2CO_3^- \rightleftharpoons H^+ + HCO_3^-$$

Lungs   Kidneys

Figure 2-30: Illustrates the acid-base balance (pH) via lungs and kidneys

The pH scale determines acid and alkaline levels. For example:

- A rise in acidity (H^+) causes pH levels to decrease.
- An increase in alkaline (basic) causes pH levels to increase.

> **Acidosis VS Alkalosis**
> - If pH is in the normal range, there is no imbalance (7.35-7.45)
> - When the levels of acid in the blood are too high, it is called acidosis as pH less than 7.35 is due to either high PCO_2 (respiratory) or low HCO_3^- (metabolic)
> - When the blood is too alkaline, it is called alkalosis. In alkaline, the pH is above 7.45, and it is due to either low PCO_2 (respiratory) or high $HCO3^-$ (metabolic).

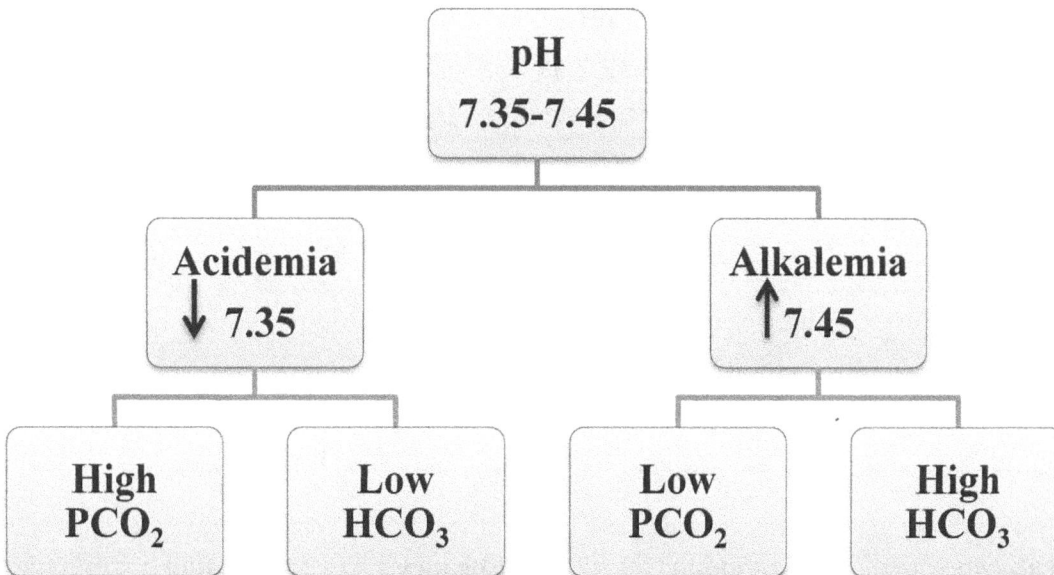

Figure 2-31: Display the Acidosis VS Alkalosis

> **Respiratory VS Metabolic**

Problems with lungs are responsible for respiratory acidosis and alkalosis.

Problems with Kidneys are responsible for metabolic acidosis and alkalosis

- **Respiratory acidosis** occurs when pH is less than 7.35 with a PCO_2 above 45. This situation manifested by tachycardia and hypotension. The treatment of choice is to increase ventilation.

- **Respiratory alkalosis** displayed by pH above 7.45 with PCO_2 less than 35, presented by shortness of breath, lightheadedness, tingling of fingertips and numbness. Treatment involves decreasing ventilation and adding dead space.

- **Metabolic acidosis** appears when pH is less than 7.35 with HCO_3^- less than 22. The sign and symptoms include vomiting and Kussmaul's respirations. The treatment of this case is to administer HCO_3^-.

- **Metabolic alkalosis** develops when pH is above 7.45 with HCO_3^- above 26. Sign and symptoms of metabolic alkalosis are weakness and hypokalemia. Treatment of choice is electrolyte therapy.

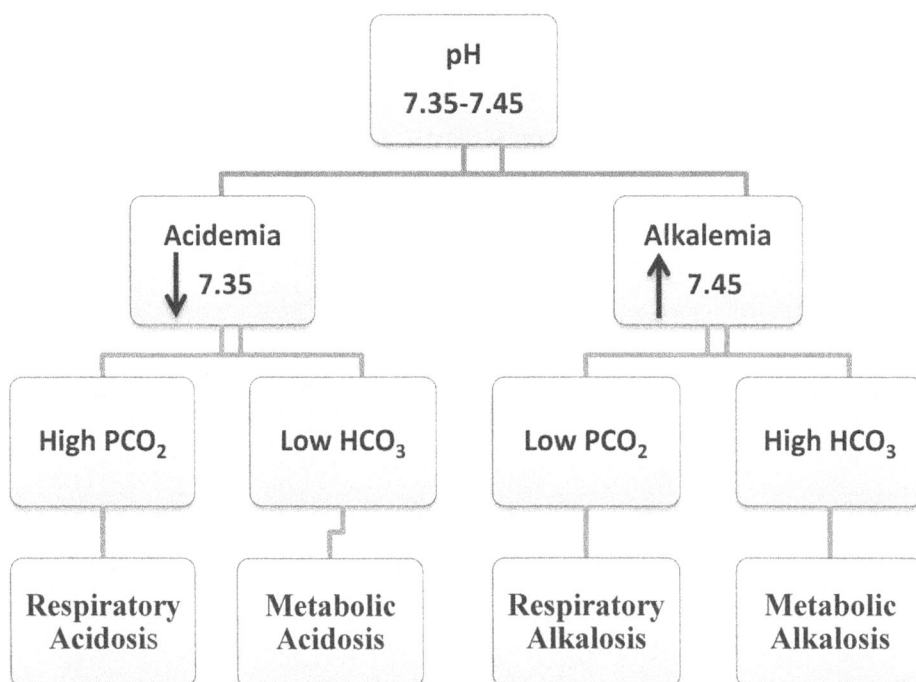

Figure 2-32: illustrates Respiratory acidosis and alkalosis (Lungs) VS Metabolic acidosis and alkalosis (Kidneys)

- ➢ **Compensated VS Uncompensated**
  - **Compensation** occurs when pH is in the normal range (7.35-7.45) while PCO_2 and HCO_3 are abnormal. This situation is typically happening in chronic cases.
  - If pH is out of range, then it is said to be **uncompensated** usually in acute cases.
- ❖ **Partial compensation** is present when both PCO2 and HCO_3^- are increased or decreased, however, pH still out of normal range. See below example:
  - o **Case: pH 7.32 (acidic)**
  - o **PCO_2 30 (low)**
  - o **HCO_3- 16 (Low)**
- ❖ **Interpretation**: partially compensated metabolic acidosis.

The following figure and table show the summary of primary and compensatory process of acid-base-balance (pH)

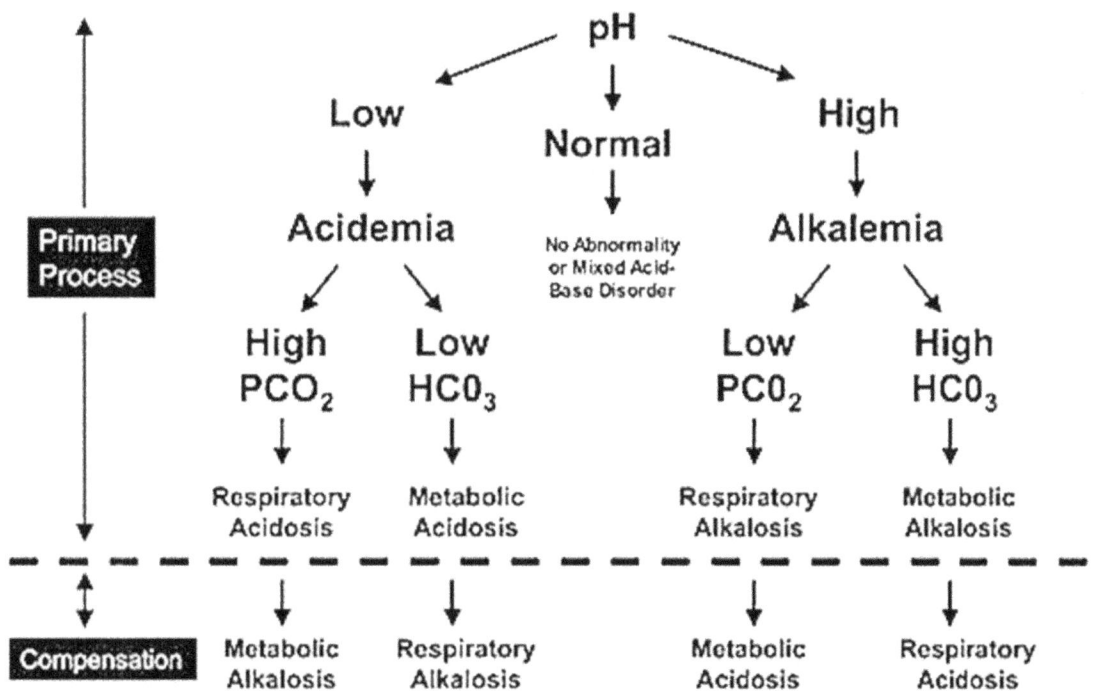

Figure 2-33: Shows the Primary and Compensatory process

Primary Event	Compensatory Event

Metabolic Acidosis

$$\downarrow pH = \frac{\downarrow HCO_3^-}{PaCO_2}$$

$$\downarrow pH = \frac{\downarrow HCO_3^-}{\downarrow PaCO_2}$$

Metabolic Alkalosis

$$\uparrow pH = \frac{\uparrow HCO_3^-}{PaCO_2}$$

$$\uparrow pH = \frac{\uparrow HCO_3^-}{\uparrow PaCO_2}$$

Respiratory Acidosis

$$\downarrow pH = \frac{HCO_3^-}{\uparrow PaCO_2}$$

$$\downarrow pH = \frac{\uparrow HCO_3^-}{\uparrow PaCO_2}$$

Respiratory Alkalosis

$$\uparrow pH = \frac{HCO_3^-}{\downarrow PaCO_2}$$

$$\uparrow pH = \frac{\downarrow HCO_3^-}{\downarrow PaCO_2}$$

Figure2-34: Illustration of The Four Primary Acid-Base Conditions and Their Compensatory Alterations

Sign and symptoms along with etiology of acid-base balance-pH (respiratory /metabolic acidosis and alkalosis are explained in a simple method as shown in figures below:

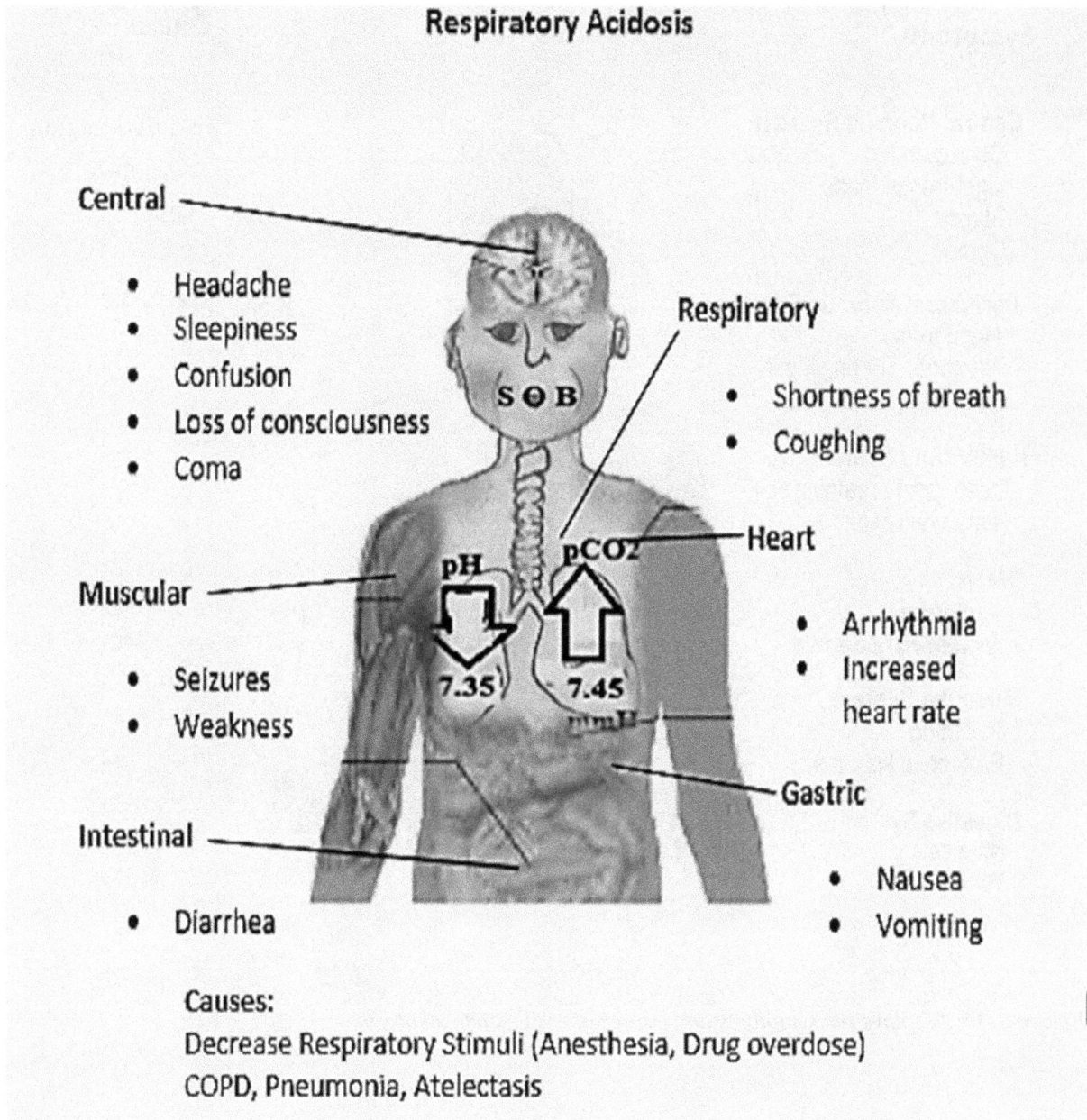

Respiratory Acidosis

Central
- Headache
- Sleepiness
- Confusion
- Loss of consciousness
- Coma

S O B

Respiratory
- Shortness of breath
- Coughing

Heart
- Arrhythmia
- Increased heart rate

Muscular
- Seizures
- Weakness

pH

pCO_2

7.35

7.45

Gastric
- Nausea
- Vomiting

Intestinal
- Diarrhea

Causes:
Decrease Respiratory Stimuli (Anesthesia, Drug overdose)
COPD, Pneumonia, Atelectasis

Figure 2-35: Displays symptoms and causes of respiratory acidosis

Respiratory Alkalosis

Symptoms

Central Nervous System
Confusion
Light-headedness
Stupor
Coma

Peripheral Nervous System
Hand tremor
Numbness or tingling in
the face, hands, or feet

Respiratory System
Deep rapid breathing
Hyperventilation

Heart
Arrhythmia
Increased heart rate

Muscular System
Twitching
Prolonged spasms

Digestive System
Nausea
Vomiting

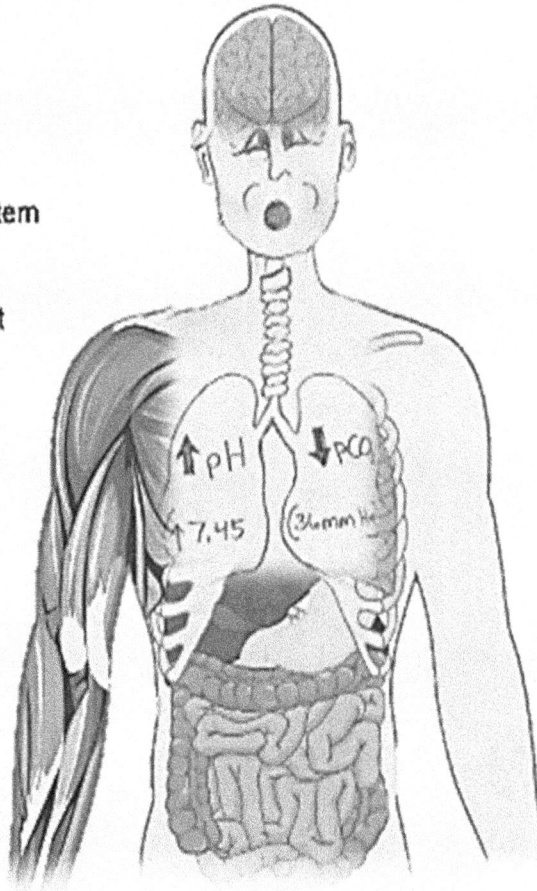

Causes

Hyperventilation
Anxiety
Fear
PE
Mechanical Ventilation

Figure 2-36: Displays the symptoms and causes of respiratory alkalosis

Metabolic Acidosis

Sign & Symptoms

CNS
- Headache
- Confusion
- Increase drowsiness

Respiratory
- Shallow Breathing
- Kussmaul Respiration

Muscular
- Twitching
- Excessive fatigue

Heart
- Decreased BP

Skin
- Flushed

Digestive system
- ↓Appetite
- Nausea
- Vomiting
- Diarrhea,

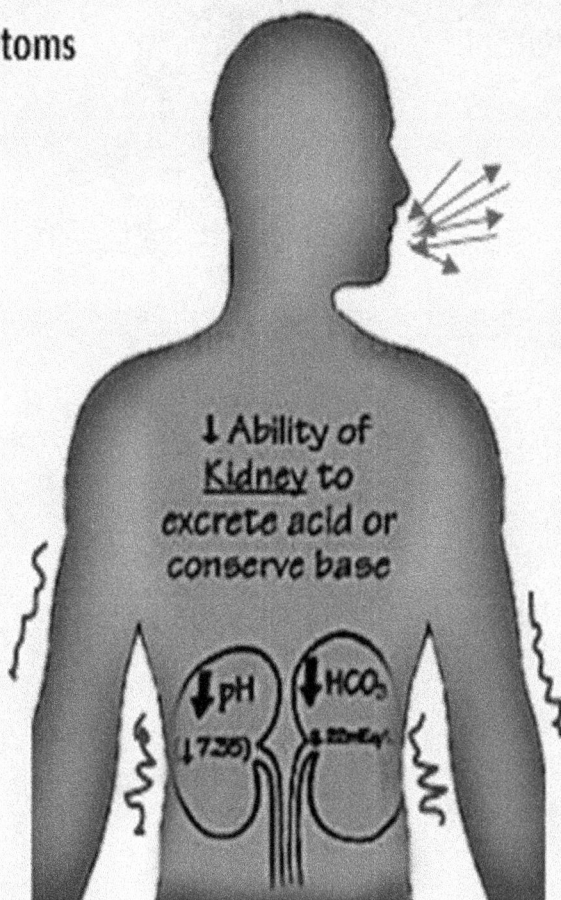

Causes
- DKA
- Severe Diarrhea
- Renal Failure
- Shock
- Aspirin poisoning
- Consumption of high fat and low carbohydrate

↓ Ability of Kidney to excrete acid or conserve base

↓pH
↓7.35)

↓HCO₃

Figure 2-37: Illustrates the signs, symptoms, and causes of Metabolic Acidosis

Metabolic Alkalosis

Sign & Symptoms

CNS
➢ Restlessness followed by lethargy
➢ Confusion
➢ Dizzy, irritable

Respiratory
➢ Compensatory Hypoventilation

Muscular
➢ Tremors
➢ Cramps
➢ Tingling of fingers and toes

Heart
➢ Dysrhythmias
➢ Tachycardia

Digestive system
➢ Nausea
➢ Vomiting
➢ Diarrhea
➢ Hypokalemia

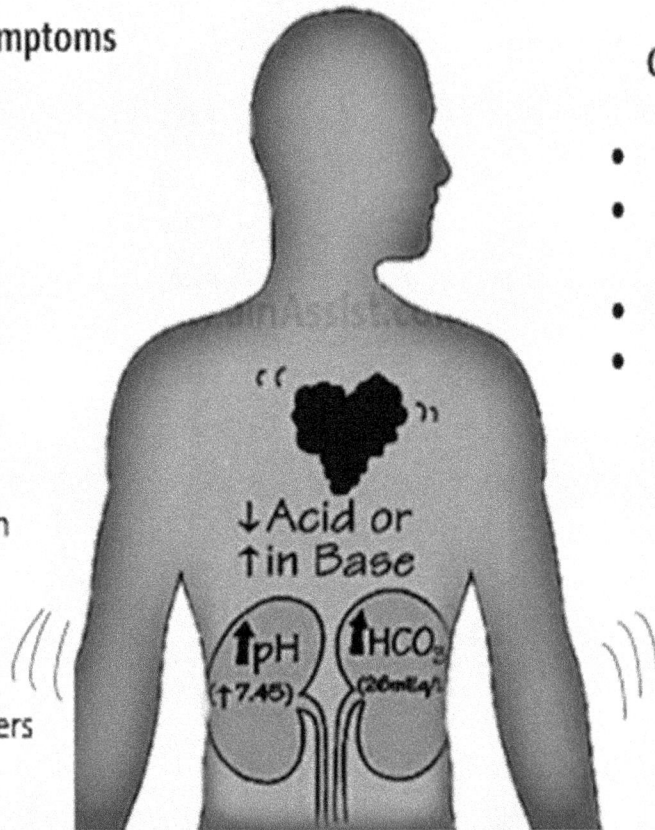

Causes
• Severe Vomiting
• Excessive GI suctioning
• Diuretics
• Excessive NaHCO3

↓Acid or ↑in Base

↑pH (↑7.45) ↑HCO₃ (26mEq/l)

Figure 2-38: Illustrates the sign, symptoms, and causes of metabolic alkalosis.

SaO$_2$- Arterial Oxygen Saturation: the percentage of the hemoglobin that is bound by oxygen. It can be calculated via blood gas analyzer or measured by noninvasive oximeter or co-oximeter. This is important to note that a significant difference between the calculated and measured values may be due to elevated carbon monoxide (COHb) levels.

Table 2-11: Displays The rule used for estimation of SaO$_2$: The "4,5,6…….7,8,9" rule.

PaO$_2$ mmHg	SaO$_2$ %
40	70
50	80
60	90

Pulmonary Function Test (PFT)

Pulmonary function tests (PFTs) are a noninvasive diagnostic procedure that provides measurable feedback about the lungs function. PFTs provide information by assessing lung volumes, capacities, rates of flow, and gas exchange; that can help in diagnosing certain lung disorders.

Certain medical conditions perhaps interfere with ventilation and may lead to chronic lung disease. These disorders are categorized as **Restrictive** or **Obstructive**:

An **obstructive** condition occurs when the air is flowing out of the lungs with difficulty causing a decreased flow of air due to resistance.

A **restrictive** disorder arises when the chest muscles are unable to expand sufficiently, generating an interruption in air flow.

Simply put, decrease lung volumes indicate a Restrictive disorder and decrease flow rates indicate an Obstructive disorder.

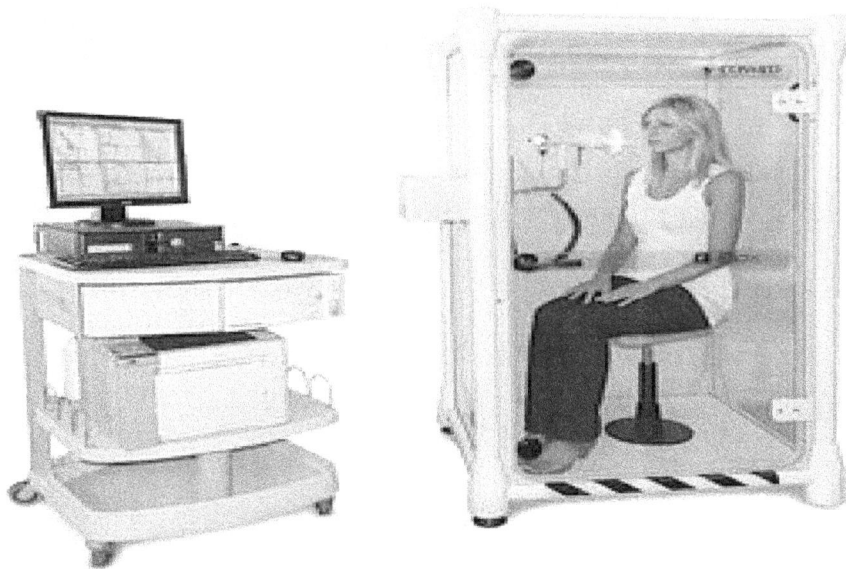

The purpose of pulmonary function tests is to

- Diagnose Obstructive (Cystic Fibrosis, Bronchitis, Asthma, Bronchiectasis, Emphysema) and restrictive (pneumonia, atelectasis, pulmonary edema) lung disease.
- Find the cause of shortness of breath (SOB)
- Measure whether lung functions is affected by exposure to chemicals at work
- Check lung function before someone has surgery
- Assess the effect of medication
- Measure progress in disease treatment

Pulmonary function tests are a comprehensive term that denotes to various procedures that measure the function of the lungs in a variety of methods. Common values that may be measured during pulmonary function testing include:

- **Tidal Volume (V_T).** The V_T is the amount of air inhaled or exhaled during normal breathing. Normal value is 500mL or 0.5 liters for male and 400-500 mL for female which is decreased with the restrictive disease. V_T * RR (Respiratory Rate) = MV (Minute Volume)

- **Vital capacity (VC).** The VC is the full volume of air that can be exhaled after maximum inspiration. Normal value 4800mL or 4.8 liters for male and 3200 mL for female which significantly decreased with restrictive disorders, therefore, it is the only volume needed to diagnose restrictive disease.

- **Functional residual capacity (FRC).** The FRC is the residual air in lungs after normal expiration. Normal value is 2400mL or 2.4 liters for male and 1800mL for female and calculated as follow: FRC = ERV + RV or FRC = TLC – IC

- **Forced vital capacity (FVC).** The FVC is the volume of air exhaled forcefully and rapidly after maximum inspiration.

- **Forced expiratory volume (FEV).** The FEV is the volume of air expired during the first, second, and third seconds of the FVC test. The most common used is FEV1, which is the only value needed to diagnose obstructive disease. The decreased value indicates obstructive abnormality and also assesses the degree of improvement after bronchodilator administration.

- **Forced expiratory flow 200-1200 (FEF $_{200-1200}$).** The average flow rate that occurs during a forced expiratory maneuver after the first 200mL has been expired. Normal value is 6L/sec. It is important to note that it measures air flow within the large airways and is decreased with mechanical problems such as tumors, obstructive disease, and poor patient effort on the FVC maneuver.

- **Forced expiratory flow 25-75% (FEF$_{25-75\%}$).** This test indicates the average rate of flow during the middle half of the FVC or forced expiratory maneuver. Normal value is 4-5 L/sec. It measures flow-rate within the small airways and decreases with obstructive disease. It is considered as the most sensitive test for detecting the presence of early small airway disease.

- **Peak Expiratory Flow Rate (PEFR)** is a measurement of the maximum volume of air during forced expiration. Normal value is 10L/sec or 600 L/minute

- **Diffusion Capacity for Carbon Monoxide (DLCO).** The DLCO Measures factors that affect diffusion of gas across the alveolar capillary membrane. Normal value is 25mlCO/min/mmHg STPD (standard temperature and pressure dry).

- **Expiratory Reserve Volume (ERV).** Expiration of the maximum volume of air from a resting end-expiratory level. Normal value 1200mL or 1.2 liters. It is decreased with the restrictive disease. It is calculated as:
  ERV = VC + IC or ERV = FRC – RV.

- **Inspiratory Capacity (IC).** The largest volume of gas that can be inspired from resting end-expiration. Typical value is 3600mL or 3.6 liters for male and 2400mL for female. It is decreased with restrictive disease and calculated as:
  IC = IRV + VT or IC = VC – ERV or IC = TLC – FRC.

- **Maximum Voluntary Ventilation (MVV).** The largest volume of air inhaled and exhaled over a 12 second period. Normal value is 170L/min. It measures the status of the respiratory muscles, compliance of the lungs and thorax as well as airway resistance. Patient efforts are estimated by multiplying the patient's FEV1 by 35; MVV less than that value indicates poor patient effort.

- **Residual Volume (RV).** The remaining volume of air in the lung at the end of maximum expiration. Typical value is 1200mL or 1.2 liter for male and 1000mL for female and calculated as follow:
  RV = FRC + ERV or RV = TLC – VC

- **Slow Vital Capacity (SVC).** Maximum expiration following a maximum inspiration. It measures V_T (Tidal volume), VC (Vital Capacity), IC (Inspiratory Capacity), ERV (Expiratory Reserve Volume) and IRV (Inspiratory Reserve Volume).

- **Total Lung Capacity (TLC).** The full volume of air in the lungs following a maximum inspiration. The typical value of TLC is 6000mL or 6.0 liter 4200mL for female.
  TLC = IRV + VT + ERV + RV
  TLC = IC + FRC
  TLC = VC + RV

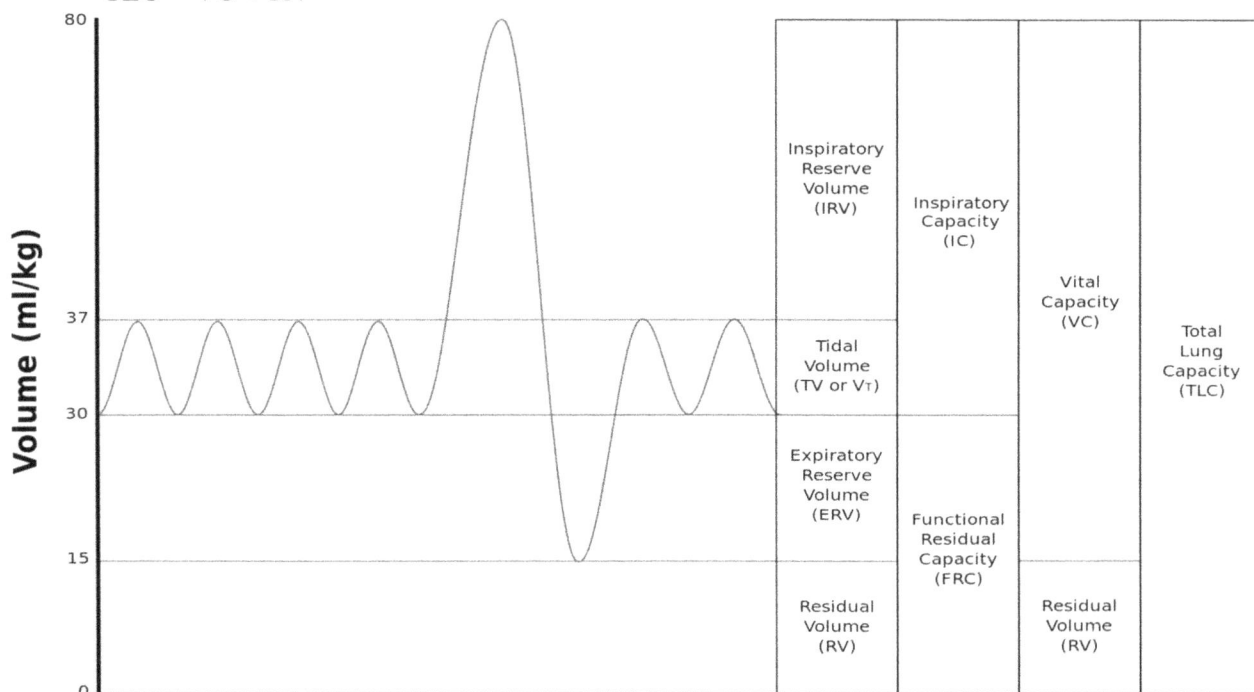

Figure 2-40: Lung Volume.jpg: Original uploader was Vihsadas at en.wikipedia derivative work: rscottweekly (https://commons.wikimedia.org/wiki/File:Lungvolumes.svg), „Lung volumes“, https://creativecommons.org/licenses/by-sa/3.0/legalcode

Factors in determining predicted value:

Age is a factor in determining predicted values. An Older individual has lower predicted values.

Height is also another important element in determining predicted values as taller patients have larger predicted values. However, the patients with spinal deformities such as Kyphoscoliosis, arm span is measured to derive the height.

Weight is not a factor in predicted values. However, it is considered in determining the presence of restrictive lung disease due to obesity.

Sex: is regarded as a factor in predicted value because females have smaller lung volumes than males.

The race is a relatively new factor in determining expected value.

There are some significant clinical histories needed before the test and interpretation of PFT results such as:

Other important elements to note are;
- **Occupational history:** type of material exposed to is important to record such as mine quarry or foundry work, mill workers, farmers, exposures to gas or fumes and dusty environment.
- **Smoking history:** is registered as pack per years. For example, if a patient has smoked two packs of cigarettes per day for the past 20 years, it would be documented as 40 pack/year smoking history. (2 X 20 = 40).
- **Medication and surgical history:** any chronic respiratory disorders such as asthma, tuberculosis, chronic bronchitis, infections or pneumonia should be noted. Any allergies and prior surgery, in particular, a pneumonectomy or lobectomy, as well as previous chest injury, should be recorded.
- **Medications:** all types of bronchodilators should be held a minimum of 4-8 hours before testing. Short-acting theophylline preparations should be held 12 hours before the test. Long-acting theophylline should be held 24 hours.
- **Vital signs**
  - Respirations: rate and pattern are of significant to note (12-20 breaths per minute).
  - Pulse: 60-100 beats per minute. The strength of pulse is significant as to note the strong and regular versus weak and thread.
  - Blood pressure: normal BP 120/80mmHg. Important to note that change in BP may be the result of increased pressures in the thorax during forced expiratory maneuvers.
  - Sensorium: the patient is required to be alert, oriented and able to follow commands. The tired, Groggy or confused patient results in an inaccurate result.

Contraindications to testing are:

- Hemoptysis in past 24 hours
- Unstable vital signs
- Unable to cooperate (sensorium)

Interpretation of the percentage predicted values displayed as follows;

- 80% or greater = normal function
- 60-79%   = mild dysfunction
- 40-59%   = moderate dysfunction
- Less than 40% = sever dysfunction

Table 2-12: Characteristic of a restrictive lung disorder in relation to lung volume and capacity

Lung Volume and Capacity	Findings
VC- Vital Capacity	↓
RV- Residual Volume	↓
FRC- Functional Residual Capacity	↓
TLC- Total Lung Capacity	↓
V_T- Tidal Volume	↓

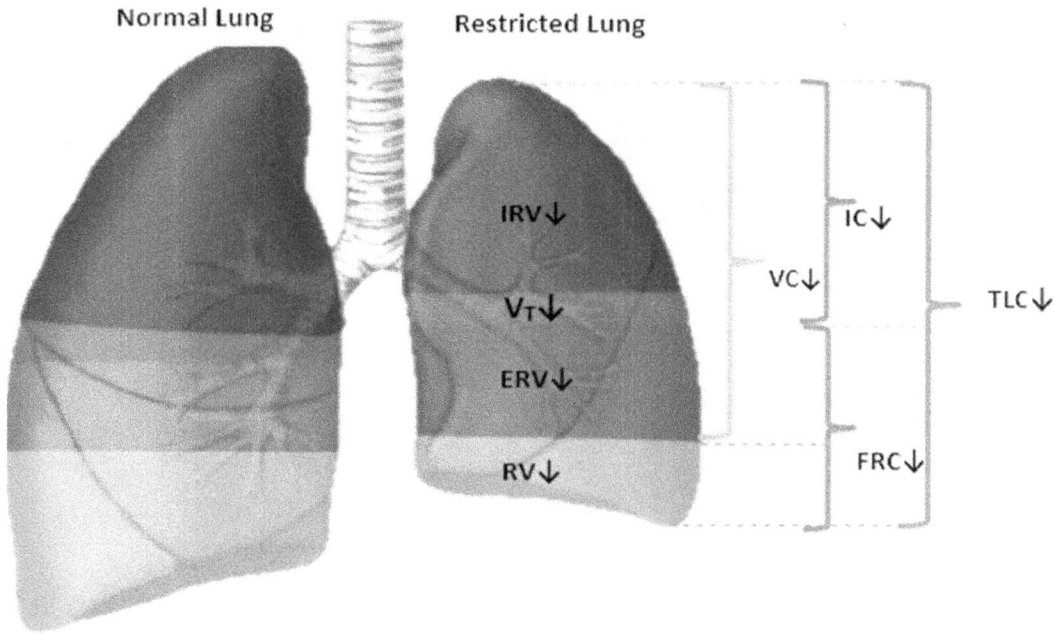

Figure 2-41: Characteristic of Restrictive Lung Disorder

The above lung volume and capacity develop in response to pathologic conditions that modify the anatomic structures distal to the terminal bronchial. These modifications causes increase lung rigidity thereby decreasing lung compliance which reduces patients VC, RV, FRC, V_T and TLC as per fig. 2-41 above.

Table 2-13: Characteristic of Obstructive Lung Disease in Relation to Lung Volume and capacity

Lung Volume and Capacity	Findings
V_T- Tidal Volume	↑
RV/TLC- Residual Volume /Total Lung Capacity Ratio	↑
RV- Residual Volume	↑
FRC- Functional Residual Capacity	↑
CV- Closing Volume	↑
VC- Vital Capacity	↓
IRV- Inspiratory Reserve Volume	↓
ERV- Expiratory Reserve Volume	↓

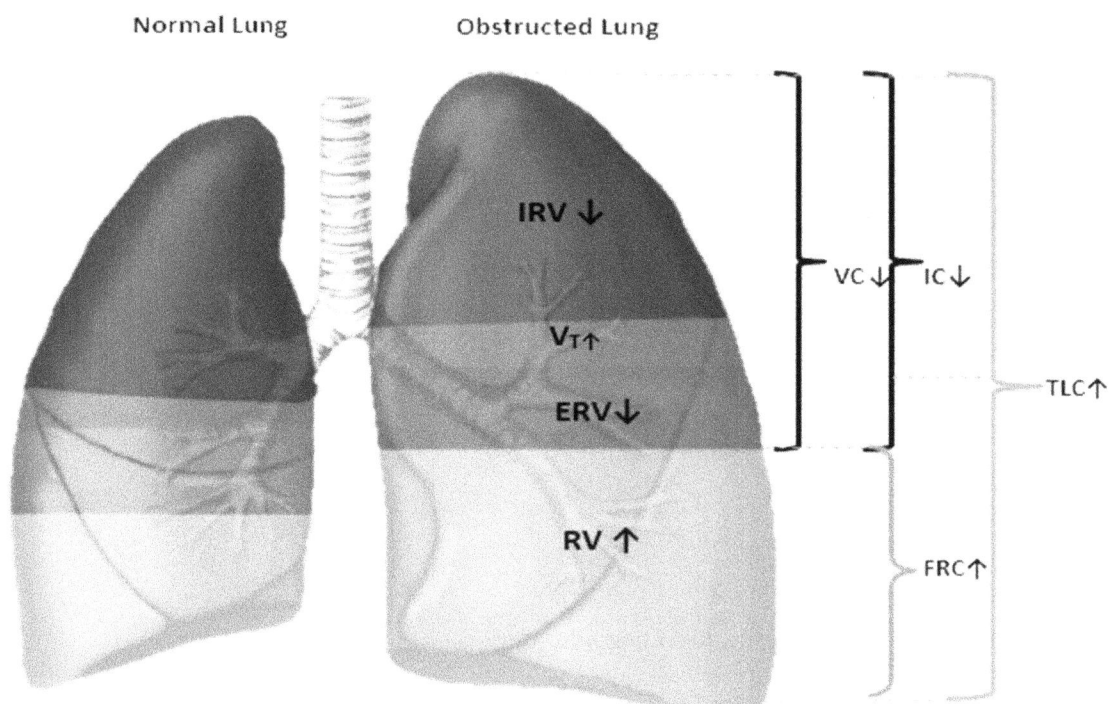

Figure 2-42: Characteristic of Obstructive Lung Disorder

The above lung volumes and capacity develop in response to pathologic conditions that alter the structures of the tracheobronchial tree resulting in increased airway resistance (R_{aw}) and during expiration causes bronchial closure. In high resistance, the patient's ventilator rate decreases and tidal volume increases to reduce work of breathing. When bronchial closure develops during expiration gas becomes trapped in alveoli and develops over distention which is called air trapping. Therefore, air trapping and bronchial closure are the major mechanisms responsible for the abnormal lung volume and capacity in obstructive pulmonary disease.

Flow Volume Loop and its Classifying Measurements

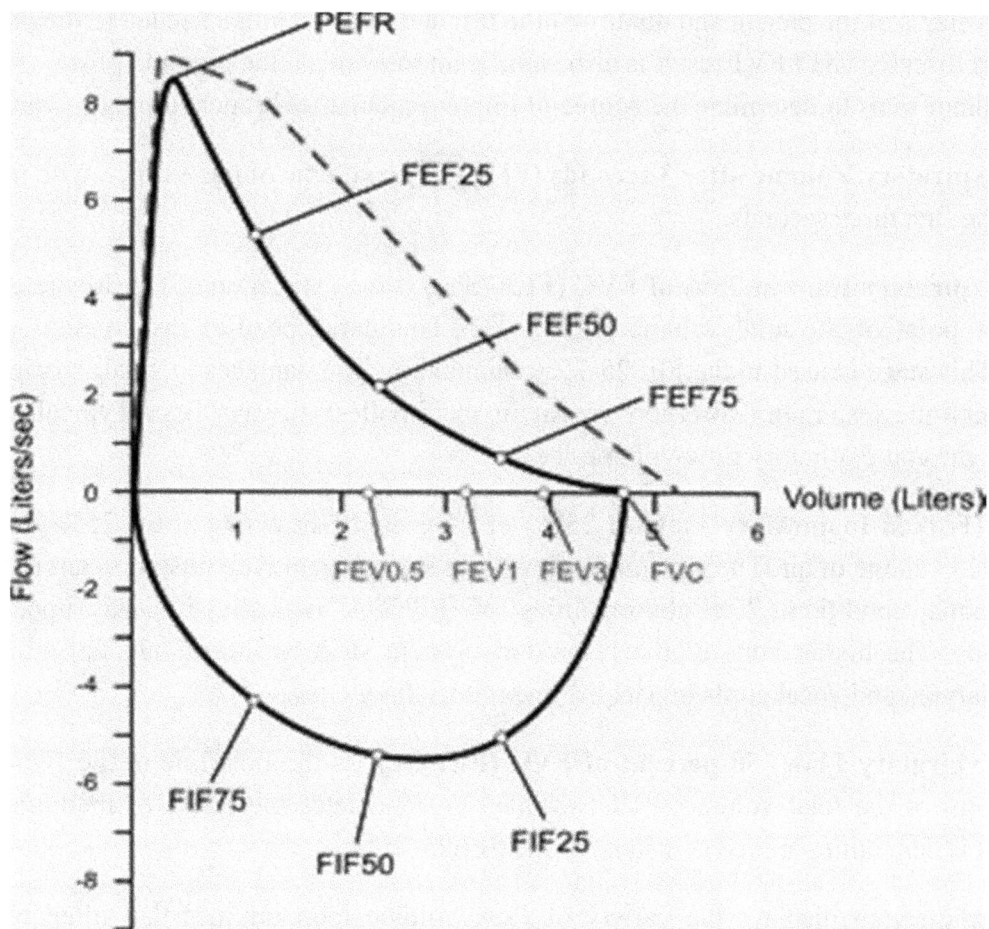

Figure 2-43: illustrates the flow volume loop and its classifying measurements. Source: http://www.morgansci.com/pulmonary-function-solutions/what-is-a-test-pulmonary-function-test/

Peak Expiratory Flow Rate (PEFR). The first explosion of air exhaled from the patient reaches this flow rate almost instantly which is the first landmark on the flow volume loop. The flow rate then rapidly slows as more air is respired. This landmark is vital in judging if the patient is giving maximal effort, the overall quality of the test, the strength of expiratory muscles, as well as the condition of the large airways (trachea and main bronchi).

Forced Expiratory Volume after half (0.5) seconds (FEV$_{0.5}$). The FEV$_{0.5}$ designates the volume of air exhaled with maximum effort in half a second.

Forced Expiratory Volume in 1 second (FEV1). The FEV1 shows the amount of air exhaled with maximum effort in the first second. The FEV1 is another important landmark in assessing the overall status of the patient and quality of the test and the only value needed to diagnose obstructive disease. The FEV1 result is also significant to evaluate the pre- and post-bronchodilator trials to determine the degree of improvement after bronchodilator administration.

Forced Expiratory Volume after 3 seconds (FEV$_3$). The volume of gas expired with maximum effort in the first three seconds.

Forced Expiratory Flow at 75% of FVC (FEF75%) is the exhalation of the flow rate at the 75 percentage point of the total volume (FVC). This landmark specifies the condition of small airways. This stage is used in the FEF25-75% calculation. The damages in small airways caused by most chronic respiratory disorders reveal in the smallest airways first. Typically, damage appears at the end-expiratory flow-volume-loop

FIF25% (Forced Inspiratory Flow at 25%) of FVC is the flow rate at the 25% point on the total inhaled volume of air. The inspiratory flow rates are comparatively insignificant in assessing the asthmatic condition. The abnormalities of FIF25% typically indicate upper airway obstructions. The higher zone of the respiratory system such as the mouth, upper and lower pharynx, larynx, and vocal cords impact the inspiratory flow rates.

Forced Expiratory Flow 50 percent of FVC (FEF$_{50\%}$). Is the flow rate of the 50% which is the midpoint of the total volume (FVC) exhaled and indicates the status of medium to small airways; it is sometimes looked at instead of the FEF25-75%.

The below diagram displays the variety of flow volume loop outlines that often relate to a particular condition. When examined in relation to the lung volume further clinical information can be revealed.

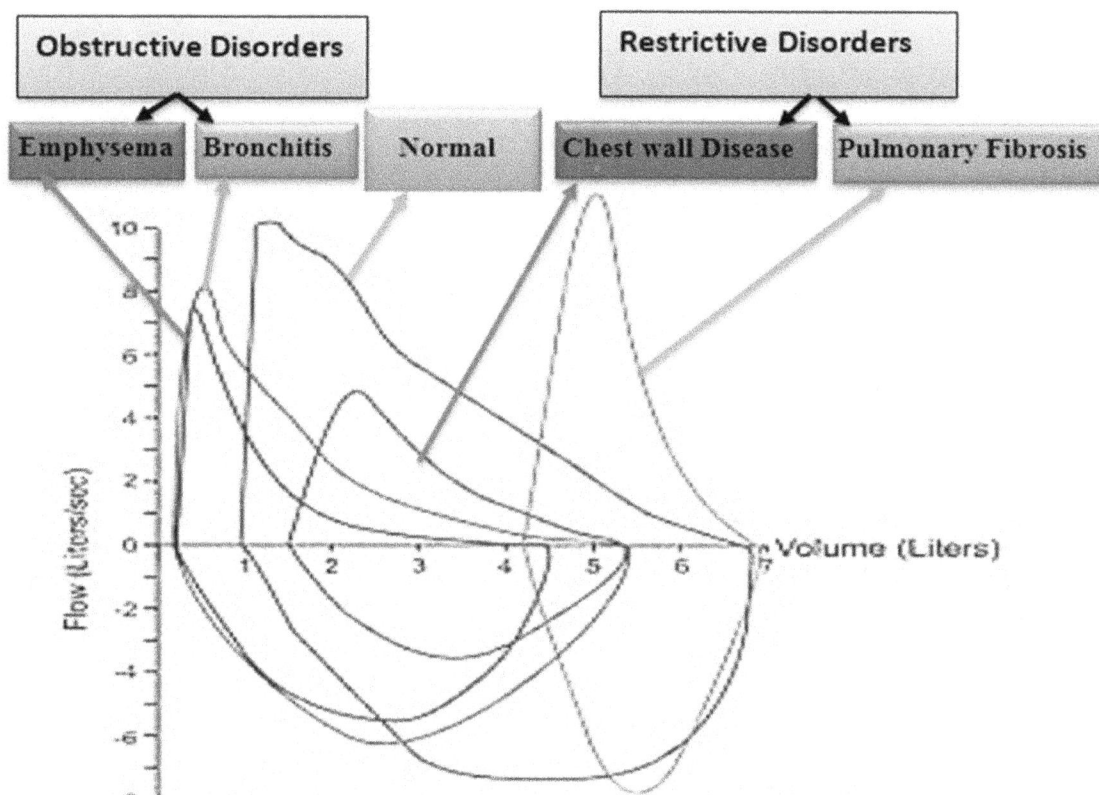

Figure 2-44: Displays the flow volume loop during obstructive and restrictive conditions

Bronchial Provocation/Methacholine Challenge Analysis

When a patient is suspected of having asthma, first spirometry is performed. If the result of the spirometry indicates no obstruction, then further testing is sometimes required. For example, a drug called **Methacholine** is used to 'provoke' airway reaction.

When the airways of patients with asthma are exposed to this drug, it stimulates a response, which can be measured. If there is a positive reaction, asthma can be clearly identified and treated applicably.

In most cases, methacholine challenge testing typically involves repeated FEV_1 efforts at increasing levels of the medication. At any stage, the patient responds by a 20% reduction in their FEV_1 compared to pre-medication, their prevalence to asthma is more likely.

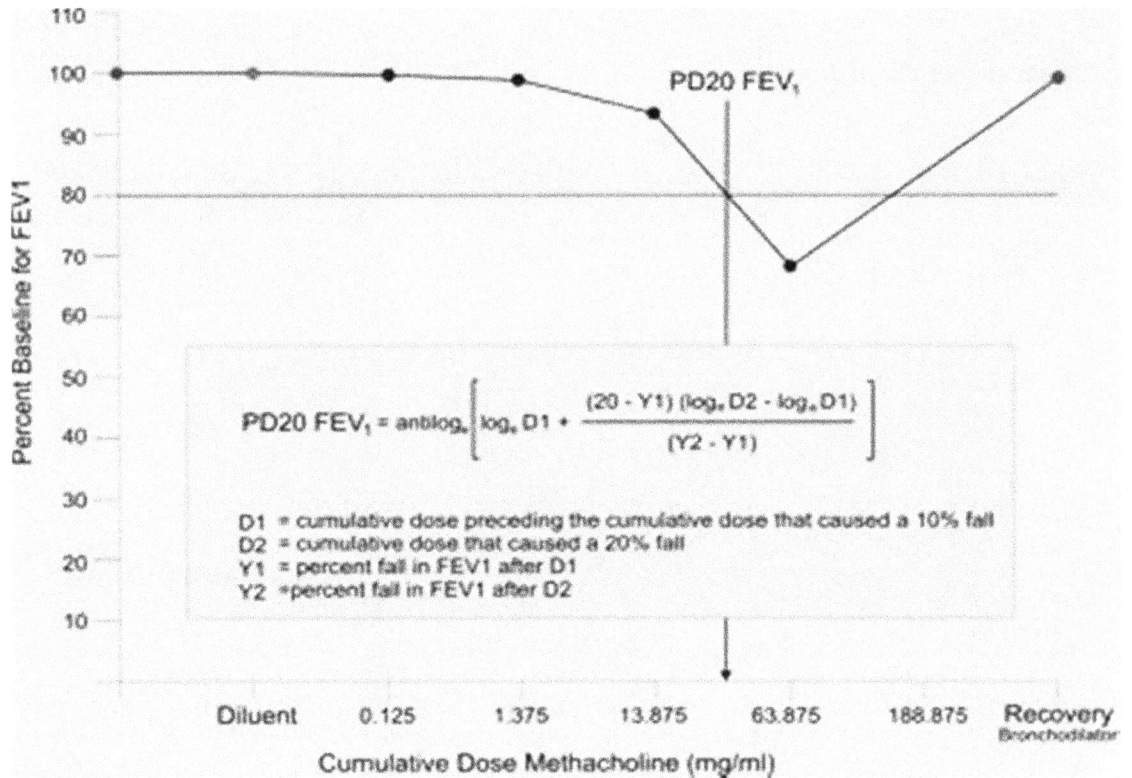

$$PD20\ FEV_1 = antilog_e \left[log_e\ D1 + \frac{(20 - Y1)\ (log_e\ D2 - log_e\ D1)}{(Y2 - Y1)} \right]$$

D1 = cumulative dose preceding the cumulative dose that caused a 10% fall
D2 = cumulative dose that caused a 20% fall
Y1 = percent fall in FEV1 after D1
Y2 = percent fall in FEV1 after D2

Figure 2-45: Illustration of methacholine challenge test in provoking airway reaction. Source:
http://www.morgansci.com/pulmonary-function-solutions/what-is-a-test-pulmonary-function-test/

Challenge testing determines the presence of airway hyperreactivity. After initial spirometry, the patient is given a specific concentration of methacholine chloride through inhalation and spirometry is repeated. Consequently, a decrease in FEV_1 by 20% below the prior test indicates asthma.

Single Breath C_O Diffusion Capacity (D_{LCO})
Measures the amount of carbon monoxide that can be inhaled and diffused across the alveolar capillary membrane into the bloodstream within a period of time.
It is reported in $mlC_O/min/mmHg$ (standard temperature and pressure dry, STPD) with normal value of 25 $mlC_O/min/mmHg$.
In testing for D_{LCO} patient exhales to residual volume, then inhales, a mixture of gas containing 0.3% C_O, 10% He and atmospheric air, rapidly to total lung capacity (TLC), hold breath for approximately 10 seconds then exhales forcefully. At the end-tidal sampler measures the concentration of gas in 1-liter sample bag.

Note: Diffusion defects are all restrictive disorders except for Emphysema (Obstructive) which is due to decreased surface area of the lungs.

Electrocardiogram (EKG) Monitoring

The EKG or ECG measures and evaluates the electrophysiology of the heart.

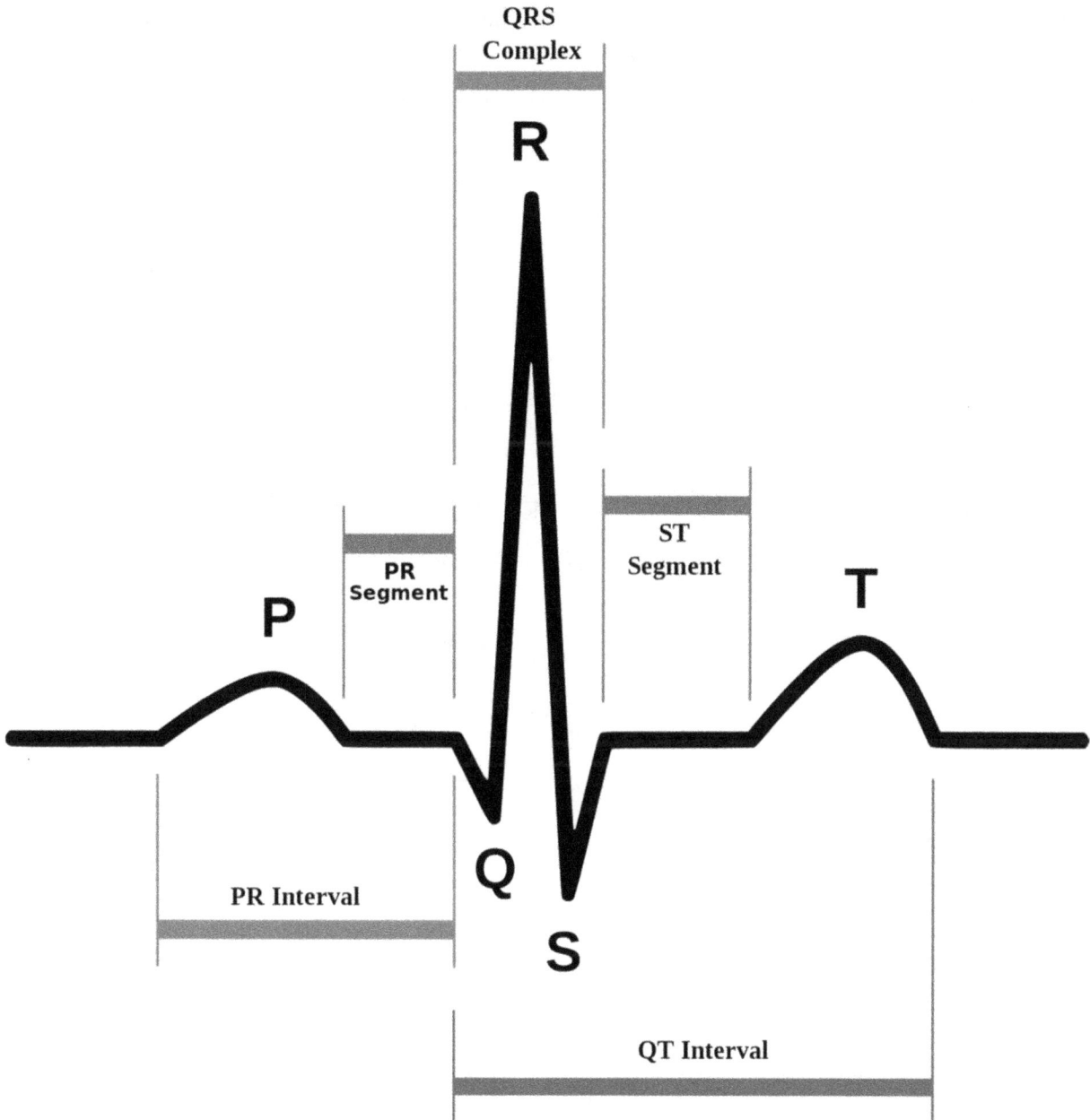

Figure 2-46: Illustrates the EKG components

The electrical impulse produced in the SA node then the wave of depolarization moves through the atria causing contraction that is called P-Wave. The impulses at that point received by the AV-node where it is delayed for a short time creating P-R interval. Impulses then continue through Bundle of His and the left and right bundle branches to the Purkinje fibers producing ventricular depolarization and contraction as QRS complex. After a short pause that is an S-T segment, the heart repolarizes as T-wave.

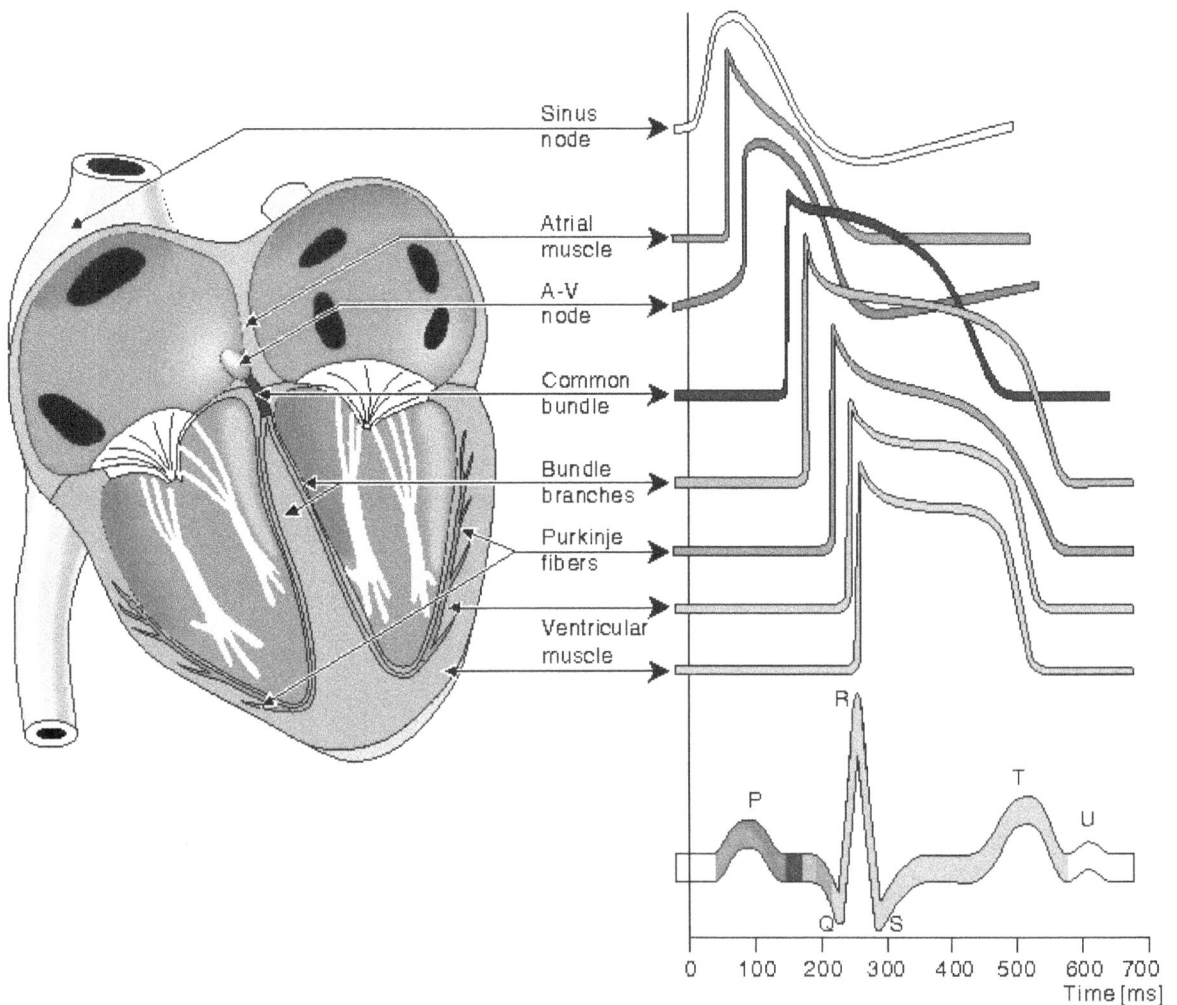

Figure 2-47: Displays the EKG Mechanism within the heart

Interpretation and management of EKG abnormalities

Table 2- 14 The Rhythm and indicated Rates

Rhythm	Rate
Normal	60-100
Bradycardia	Less than 60
Tachycardia	Greater than 100
Flutter	Greater than 200
Fibrillation	Too fast to count

Fibrillation and Flutter can be either atrial or ventricular. Ventricular fibrillation is life threatening.

The rate of an EKG can be estimated by measuring the distance between two R waves.

- Standard Rate: The distance between the two R waves is 3 to 5 large blocks.
- Bradycardia: the distance between the two R-waves is wider than five large blocks then the rate is less than 60.
- Tachycardia: The distance between the two R-waves are closer than three large blocks then the rate is greater than 100.

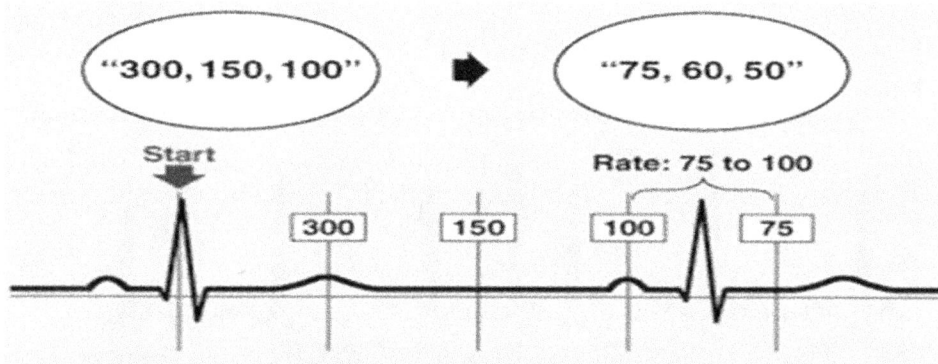

Figure 2-48: Illustrates the EKG measurement of the distance between the two R waves.

Heart Rate calculated via dividing 300 by the number of large blocks between R waves.

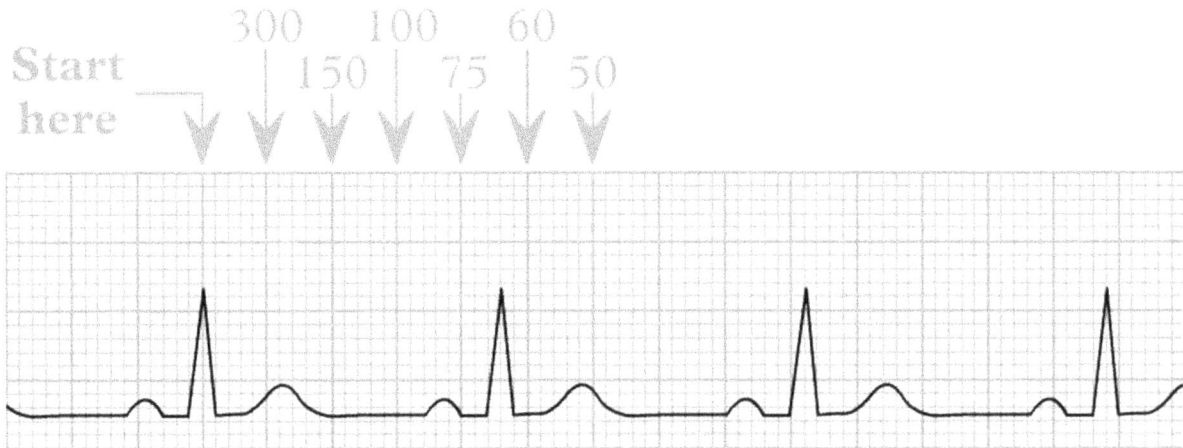

Figure 2-49: Shows the calculation of the heart rate via number of large blocks

Arrhythmias

An arrhythmia is an irregular heartbeat – a problem with the rate and rhythm of the heartbeat. The heart may beat excessively fast called tachycardia, or it may beat too slow as it known as bradycardia, too early (premature contraction) or too irregularly (fibrillation). Arrhythmias are heart rhythm problems; they arise when the electrical impulses in the heart that coordinate heartbeats are not functioning properly, making the heart beat too fast/slow or inconsistent.

- **Normal Sinus Rhythm (NSR):** Normal rate with no skip or extra beats. Require no treatment. See figure below:

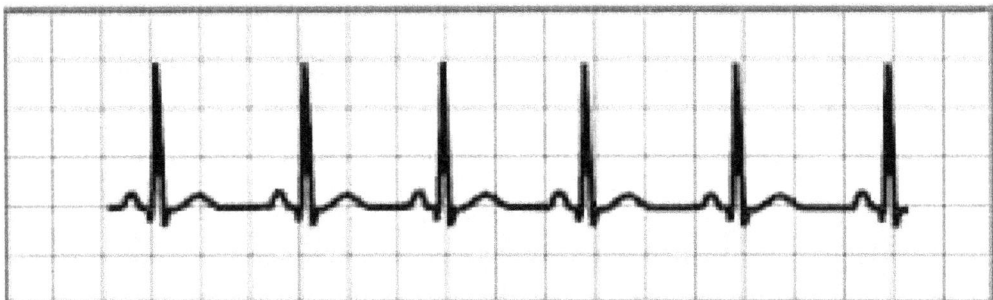

Figure 2-50 shows the normal sinus rhythm

- **Sinus Bradycardia** illustrated by a sinus rhythm with a rate of less than 60 requires treatment with atropine/epinephrine as seen in the following illustration:

SINUS BRADYCARDIA
Impulses originate at S-A node at slow rate

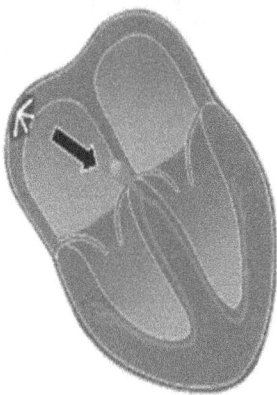

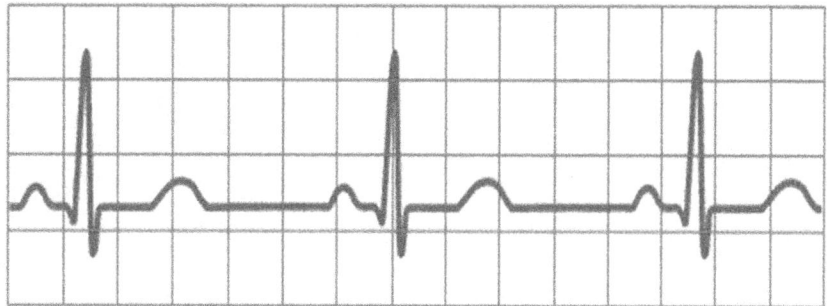

All complexes normal, evenly spaced. Rate < 60/min.

Figure 2-51: shows the Sinus Bradycardia

- **Sinus Tachycardia** is a sinus rhythm with rate > 100 requires treating the symptoms.

SINUS TACHYCARDIA
Impulses originate at S-A node at rapid rate

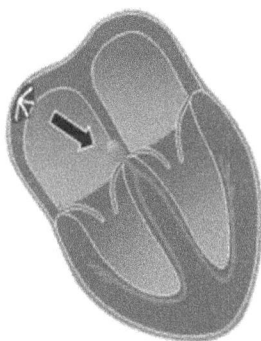

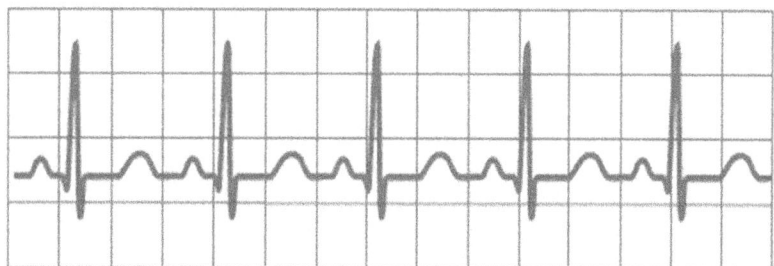

All complexes normal, evenly spaced. Rate >100/min.

Figure 2-52: shows Sinus Tachycardia

- **Premature ventricular contractions PVC's**: treated with Lidocaine and oxygen. See figure below:

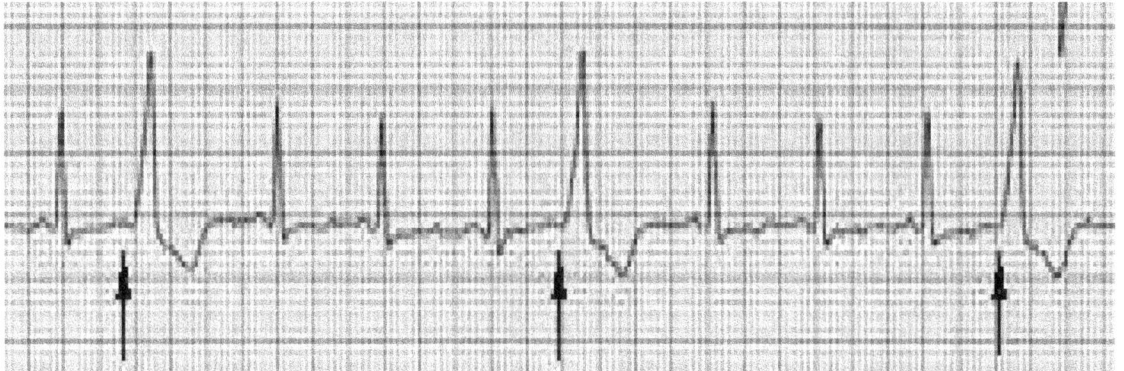

Figure 2-53: shows PVC

- **Ventricular Tachycardia** - V-Tach, ventricular rhythm with rate > 100. If there is no pulse the treatment requires defibrillation with 200 joules.

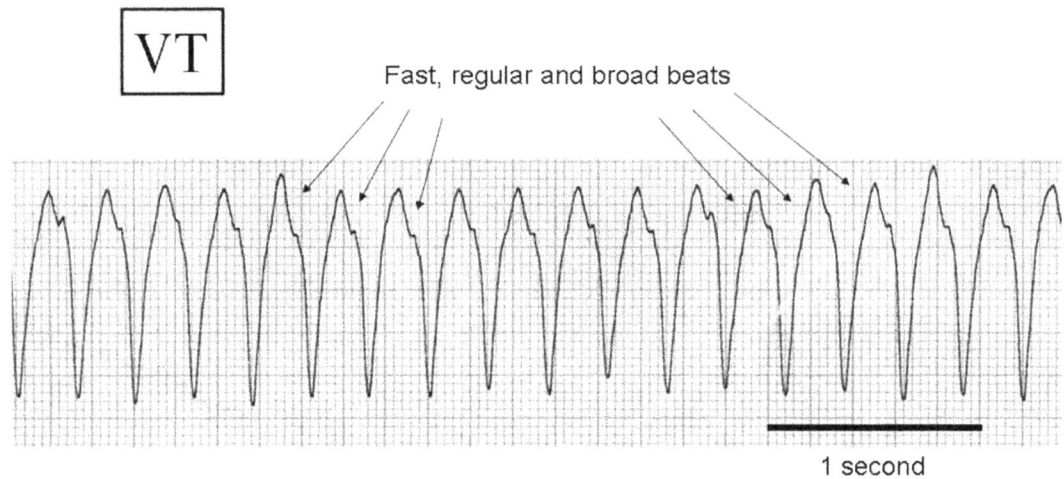

Figure 2-54: Displays Ventricular Tachycardia rhythm

- **Ventricular Fibrillation** – V-Fib, completely irregular ventricle rhythm. Rate and rhythm cannot be determined.

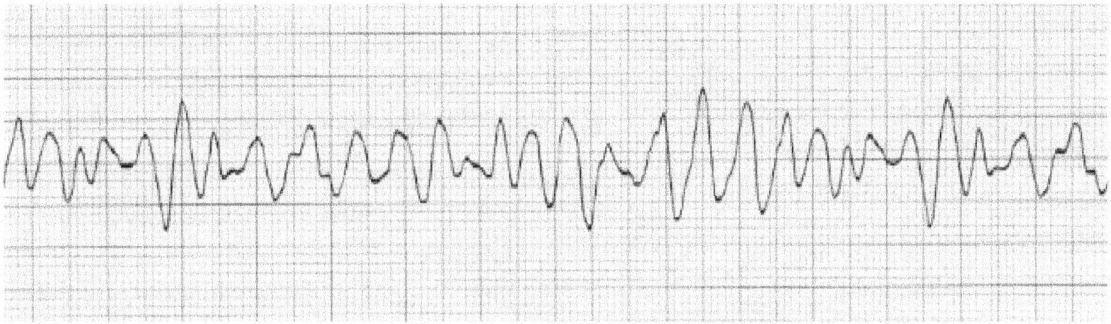

A severely abnormal heart rhythm (arrhythmia) that can be life-threatening.
Emergency- requires Basic Life Support
Rate cannot be discerned, rhythm unorganized

Figure 2-55: Shows Ventricular Fibrillation rhythm

The cardiac arrest involving V-tach and V-fib treatment algorithm is presented in the figure 2-56 shown below.

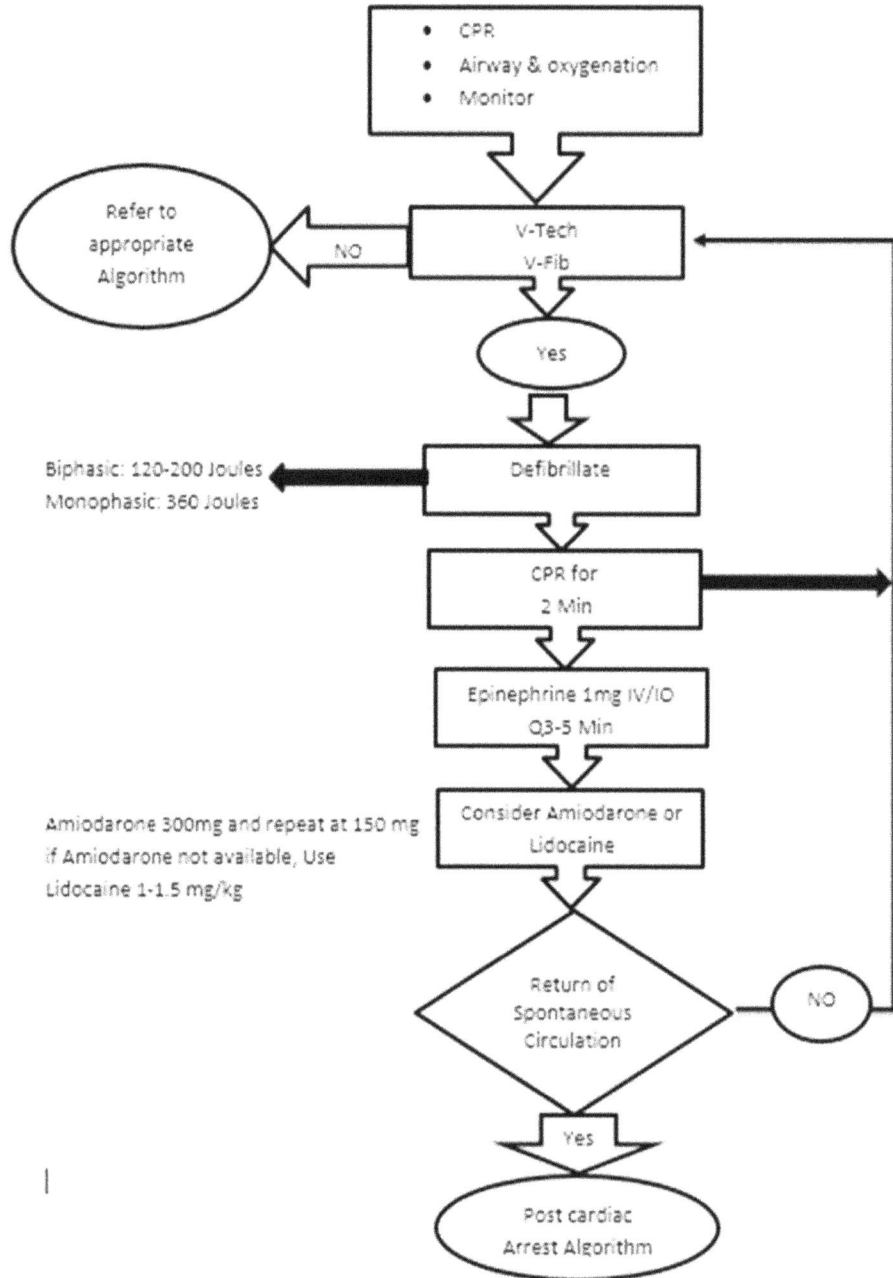

Figure 2-56 Illustrates the algorithm of cardiac arrest: VT and V. Fib

1.   What is meant by life functions?

2.   Explain ways to perform the chest assessment.

3.   Describe the Ventilatory-Perfusion ratio.

4.   Describe the process of ventilation regulation.

5.   Explain the mechanism of Pulmonary Shunt.

6.   Describe the lung compliance and its effect on ventilation process.

7.   Describe airway resistance and its effect on ventilation process.

8.   Explain the cough and sputum production mechanism.

9.   Describe Polycythemia, Core-Pulmonale.

10.   Explain the importance of Arterial Blood Gasses and its process.

11.   Explain the Pulmonary Function Test (PFT) and its process

12.   Explain the Electrocardiogram (ECG, EKG) and its use.

Subsequent Chapters

Common Respiratory Disorders

- Chronic Chough
- Asthma
- Chronic Bronchitis
- Emphysema
- COPD
- Bronchiectasis
- Pneumonia
- Pulmonary Edema
- ARDS
- Flail Chest
- Pneumothorax
- Pleural Effusion
- Pulmonary Embolism
- Tuberculosis
- Croup Syndrome
- Cystic Fibrosis
- Sleep Apnea
- Lung Cancer

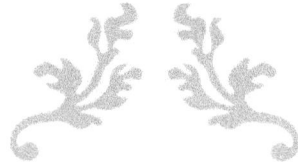

Chapter 3
Chronic Chough

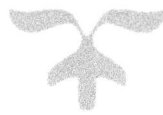

Chapter Objectives

1. Description of chronic cough
2. Describe the mechanism of chronic cough
3. Explain the etiologic factors of chronic cough
4. Treatment options for chronic cough

Chronic Cough

A cough that persists over time, eight weeks or longer in adult and four weeks in children, is called chronic cough. A chronic cough is not only an aggravation but also interrupts sleep and cause exhaustion, vomiting, dizziness and in severe cases rib fracture. A chronic cough is a common problem and is not considered a disease, but rather a symptom of an underlying disorder.

There are numerous variation forms of a persistent cough as listed below:

- **A chronic dry cough:** is a cough that causes irritation of lungs and throat and does not produce any mucus. Most likely, it is the sign of viral infection or sinus condition.
- **A persistent wet cough** produces mucus that depending on the color of the sputum possible indication of a bacterial infection or fluid in the lungs such as congestive heart failure.
- **A stress cough**: stress causes a reflexive spasm of the airways. A stress cough does not produce mucus and is not typically related to infections.
- **A barking cough**: it is usually a childhood condition such as croup or other viral disorder.
- **A harsh barking cough**: is caused by inflammation of trachea.
- **A whooping cough or pertussis** is a highly contagious respiratory disease and can be lethal for children under one year of age.

Mechanism of Cough

- Initiates with a gasp causing air to be drawn into the lungs
- Epiglottis closes the trachea
- Forceful contraction of Abdominal muscles, diaphragm and chest
- Pressure builds up in the lungs and airways
- Epiglottis is opened
- Blast of air is released forcefully
- Cough sound

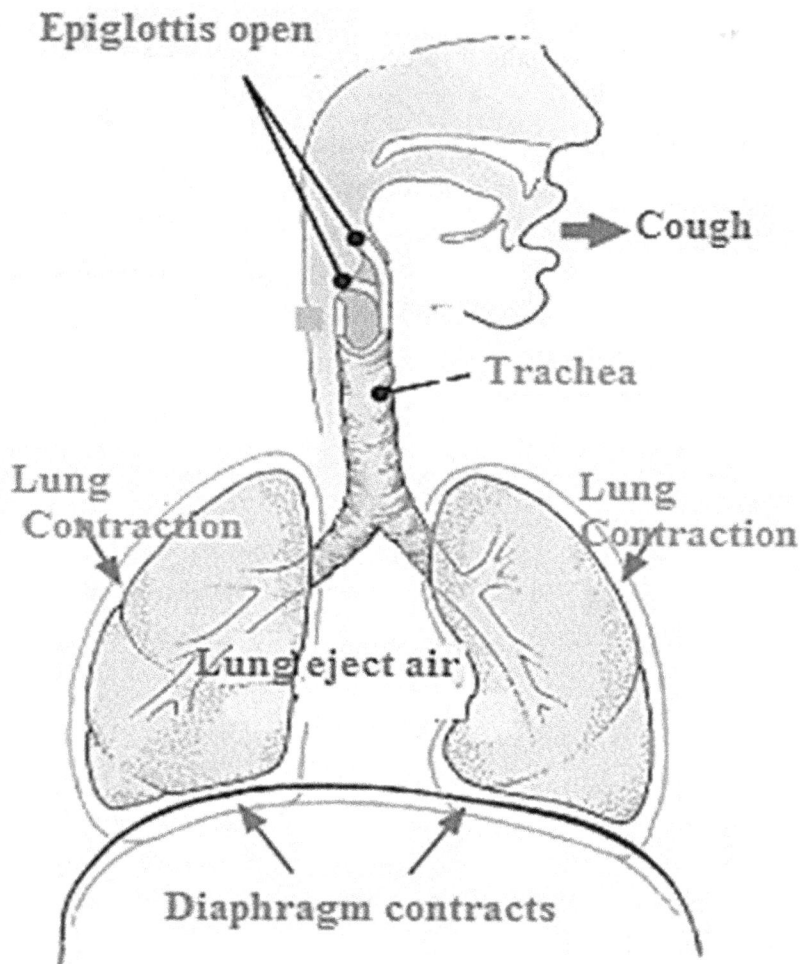

Figure 3-1 Illustrates the cough mechanism

Etiologic Factors of a Chronic Cough

The common contributing factors of a chronic cough are listed below:

- Tobacco smoking is one of the most causative factors of persistent chronic cough.
- Asthma disorder results in wheezing, breathing difficulty, and chronic cough that is typically aggravated by cold air, pollutants, pollen, smoke, and odor.
- Acid Reflux or Gastroesophageal Reflux Disease (GERD) is the backward flow of the stomach content into the esophagus and airway that result in airway spasm, shortness of breath and cough.
- Sinus congestion and post nasal drip cause a chronic cough. The symptom initiates with a tickle or scratchy throat with frequent throat clearing.

- Bacterial or viral or fungal infections can cause an acute or a chronic cough. For example, bronchitis and pneumonia, tuberculosis, upper respiratory infection, cold and flu often produce a cough.
- Pertussis or whooping cough condition is a highly contagious respiratory infection caused by Bordetella pertussis causing a forceful, rapid, and continuous cough that can be fatal in children.
- Foreign objects obstructing the airways can cause a cough.
- Some medications such as ACE inhibitor in treating hypertension can cause a chronic cough. Among those medications are Vasotec (enalapril), Capoten (captopril).
- Other causes of a chronic cough include allergies, tumors, sarcoidosis, chronic obstructive pulmonary disease (COPD) congestive heart failure (CHF) and emphysema.

Treatment of Chronic Cough

The initial treatment is to encourage patients to cease smoking and to avoid second-hand smoke since the continuation of the use of tobacco smoke will deteriorate the lungs further. The majority of patients with a chronic cough will no longer cough after one month of smoking cessation.

The etiologic factor of a cough typically determines the treatment. A chronic cough resulting from medication and disorders are treated as follow:

- Asthma condition that results in a persistent cough are treated with inhaled bronchodilators and inhaled steroids, or in some cases, short-term oral steroids are given to relieve a chronic cough.
  Relievers are bronchodilator drugs that relieve the symptoms of asthma such as a cough, chest tightness, breathlessness, and wheezing. The relievers are classified as Sympathomimetic (adrenergic), Parasympathetic (anticholinergics) and Xanthine bronchodilators.

Sympathomimetic Mechanism of Action
  ➢ Direct $\beta 2$ stimulation, stimulate adenyl cyclase that increase cAMP thereby results in bronchodilation.
  ➢ Inhibits mediators release from mast cells.
  ➢ Increases ciliary activity resulting in increased mucus clearance
Sympathomimetic drugs are classified into selective $\beta 2$-agonists and non-selective β-agonists as shown in Table 3-1.

Table 3-1 Classification of Sympathomimetic drugs

Selective β2-agonists	Non-selective β-agonists

Short Acting β2-agonists
• **Salbutamol (albuterol, Ventolin) inhalation, orally and I.V.**
• **Terbutaline given via inhalation, orally and S.C.**
• **levalbuterol (Xopenex))**
• **pirbuterol (Maxair)**
 	
➢ **Rapid onset of action 15-30 min**
➢ **Duration of action 4-6 hr.**
➢ **For acute asthmatic episode**
 	
Long Acting β2-agonists
• **Salmeterol (Serevent, inhalation)**
• **Formoterol (Foradil, inhalation)**
  ➢ **Long-acting bronchodilator 12hrs**
  ➢ **Low onset of action**
  ➢ **Not used for acute episodes**
  ➢ **Used for prophylaxis as nocturnal asthma**
  ➢ **Combined with inhaled corticosteroids to control asthma**
• **Advantages of β2-agonists**
  ➢ **Minimal CVS side effect**
  ➢ **Appropriate for asthmatic patients with hypertension or heart conditions**
• **Disadvantages of β2-agonists**
  ➢ **Skeletal muscle tremors**
  ➢ **Nervousness**
  ➢ **Tachycardia**
	Epinephrine (isoprenaline)
	➢ Potent Bronchodilator
	➢ Rapid Action within 15 minutes
	➢ Aerosol Nebulizer or S.C. delivery
	➢ Duration of action 60-90 minutes
	➢ Drug of choice for acute anaphylaxis
	
	• **Disadvantages**
	  ➢ Not effective orally
	  ➢ Hyperglycemia in diabetes
	  ➢ CVS side effect: tachycardia, arrhythmia, hypertension and angina
	  ➢ Skeletal muscle tremor

Parasympatholytic (anticholinergic) agents also called Muscarinic antagonists
This agent inhibits bronchoconstriction and mucus secretion. Medications are used for acute severe asthma combined with β2-agonists and steroids. A most popular example of a non-selective muscarinic antagonist is ipratropium bromide or Atrovent and tiotropium or Spiriva administered via aerosol inhalation.

- **ipratropium bromide (Atrovent)**
- **tiotropium (Spiriva)**

- ➤ A short-acting bronchodilator
- ➤ Less effective than β2-agonists
- ➤ No anti-inflammatory action
- ➤ Minimal systemic side effects

Methyl-xanthine or xanthine bronchodilators
Xanthine are used to enhance bronchial smooth muscle relaxation
- ➤ Theophylline is given orally and parenterally
- ➤ Aminophylline (combination of theophylline and ethylenediamine) given orally and parenterally.

Mechanism of action
- ➤ Phosphodiesterase inhibitors
- ➤ ↑cAMP results in bronchodilation
- ➤ Adenosine receptors antagonists (A1)
- ➤ Increase diaphragmatic contraction
- ➤ Improves ventilation
- ➤ Stabilizes mast cell membrane

- GERD cause of a chronic cough is initially treated with avoiding food that increases reflux, avoiding food before bedtime, elevating the head of the bed while sleeping. The medications commonly prescribed for the treatment of GERD are listed in Table 3-2

Table 3-2 List of medication for the treatment of GERD

Generic	Brand
famotidine	Pepcid
cimetidine	Tagamet
ranitidine	Zantac
omeprazole	Prilosec
lansoprazole	Prevacid
rabeprazole	Aciphex
pantoprazole	Protonix
esomeprazole	Nexium

- Sinus congestion and post-nasal drip:
  - ➤ Use of nasal decongestants such as Sudafed (pseudoephedrine) and
  - ➤ Antihistamines such as Benadryl (diphenhydramine)
  - ➤ Inhaled nasal steroids in treating rhinitis
  - ➤ Atrovent (ipratropium bromide) Nasal inhalers

- Microbial infections
  Bacterial infections such as bronchitis and pneumonia are typically treated with antibiotics such as cephalosporins, azithromycin.

Table 3-3 List of antibiotics used to treat bacterial infections

Fluoroquinolones	Macrolides	Sulfonamides	Tetracyclines
levofloxacin (Levaquin)	clarithromycin (Biaxin) azithromycin (Zithromax and Zmax)	sulfamethoxazole and trimethoprim (Bactrim)	doxycycline (Vibramycin)

- ACE inhibitors known to cause a chronic cough should switch to the new generation of ACE inhibitor called ARBs (angiotensin receptor blockers) such as:
  - ➢ Diovan (valsartan)
  - ➢ Cozaar (losartan)

- **Cough suppressants and Expectorants**

These agents are used to comfort patients by reducing the cough and reduce mucus viscosity to facilitate the mobilization and expectoration of bronchial secretions. Table 3-3

Table 3-4. List of cough suppressants and expectorants

dextromethorphan Cough suppressants	guaifenesin Expectorants
Pertussin	Robitussin
Vicks 44	Mucinex
Benylin	

- Severe cases of a chronic cough are treated by prescribing codeine and similar narcotic drugs that are effective cough suppressants.

- A chronic cough can sometimes be treated with home remedies as follows:
  - ➢ Head elevation with extra pillows at night to ease a chronic cough
  - ➢ Do not smoke tobacco products and avoid inhaled irritants such as smoke, dust, or other pollutants.
  - ➢ Staying hydrated by drinking sufficient amount of water
  - ➢ gargling with warm salt water, to loosen the mucus
  - ➢ cough drops, cough lozenges to soothe a sore throat
  - ➢ Inhaling steam
  - ➢ Ginger and honey as prepared tea to relieve the cough symptoms
  - ➢ A persistent cough are often relieved with Eucalyptus or mint

1. What is a chronic cough?

2. List the different forms of a persistent cough.

3. Explain the role of cigarette smoking in a chronic cough.

4. Provide the etiologic factors of a chronic cough.

5. List the medications commonly used in the treatment of a chronic cough.

6. List the home remedies that can be used to aid in treating chronic cough.

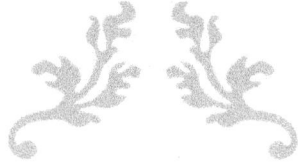

Chapter 4

Asthma

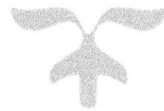

Chapter Objectives

1. Description of asthma
2. Explain the Pathologic Changes of the lungs during asthma
3. Identify common symptoms of asthma
4. Explain etiologic factors of asthma
5. Performing chest assessment and diagnostic findings
6. Treatment options for asthma

Asthma

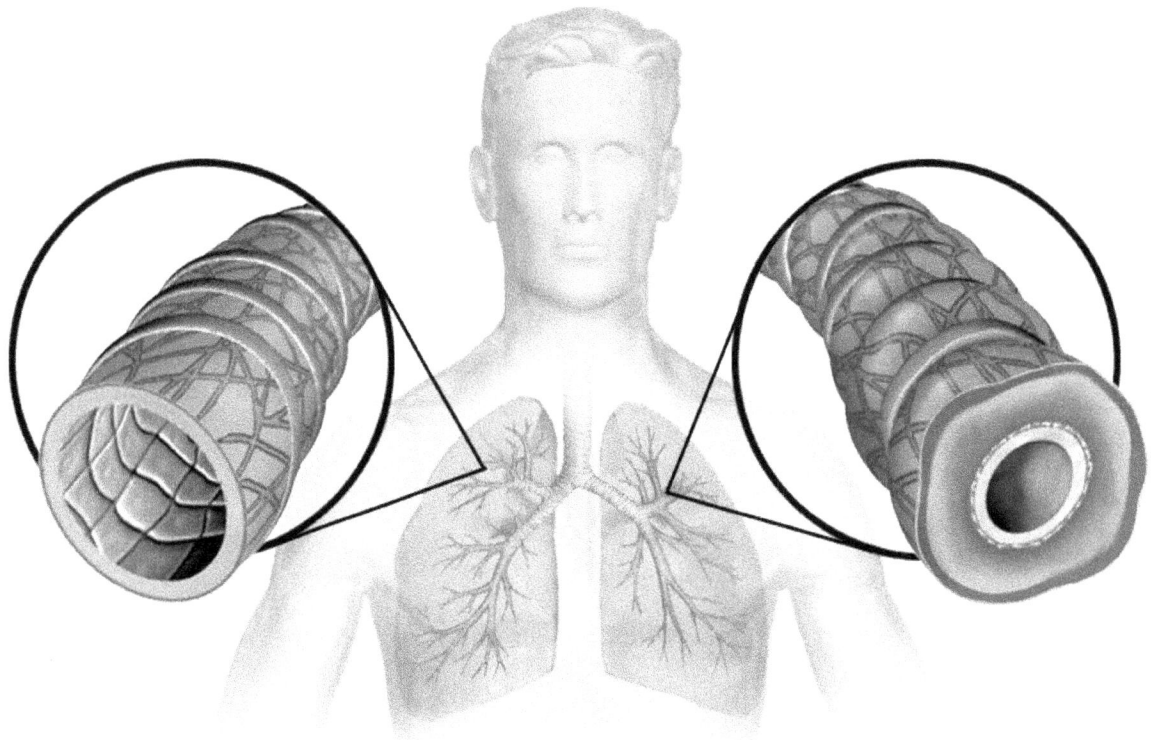

Figure 4-1: Illustration of Pre and post asthma episode. Source: BruceBlaus(https://commons.wikimedia.org/wiki/File:Asthma_(Lungs).png), https://creativecommons.org/licenses/by-sa/4.0/

Asthma

Asthma is a chronic lung disorder causing constriction of the airway muscles and inflammation of the airways. Asthma causes repeated episodes of coughing often transpires at night or early morning, Shortness of breath (SOB), wheezing, chest tightness. Asthma affects people of all ages and ethnicity; however, it is the most common chronic ailment of childhood. Among children, asthma is about two times more prevalent in boys than girls. However, after puberty, asthma episode is more frequent in girls.

Pathologic Changes of the Lungs

During an asthma attack, the lungs undergo the following changes:

- Constriction of the smooth muscles surrounding the small airways in response to a particular stimulus.
- Hypertrophy of smooth muscle layers up to three times their normal size.
- The proliferation of goblet cells.
- Enlargement of bronchial mucous glands.
- Production of thick, tenacious mucus and extensive mucus plugging may develop in the airways.
- The bronchial mucosa is edematous and infiltrated with eosinophils.
- The cilia become damaged.
- The basement membrane of the mucosa becomes thicker than normal.
- Develop air trapping and alveolar hyperinflation

A notable feature of bronchial asthma is that the anatomic alterations that occur during an asthma attack are completely absent between the asthmatic episodes.

To recapitulate, the main anatomic alteration during an asthmatic event are as follows:

- Smooth muscle constriction of bronchial airways
- Excessive production of thick, tenacious tracheobronchial secretions
- Hyperinflation of alveoli

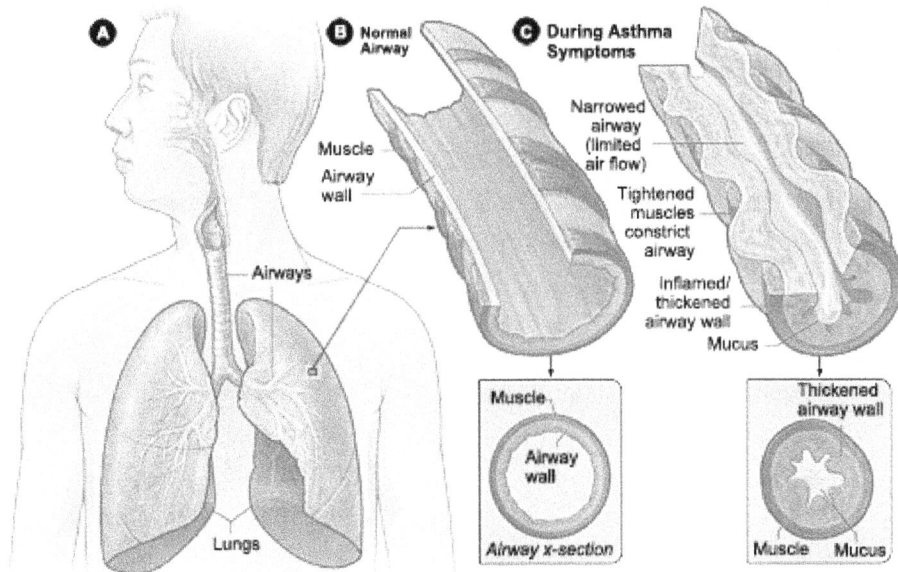

Figure 4-2: (A) shows the position of the lungs and airways in the body. (B) displays a cross-section of a normal airway. (C) Shows a cross-section of an airway during an asthma attack. Source: Google images labeled for reuse; en.wikipedia.org (Public Domain)

Most Common Visible Symptoms of Asthma

(for physiologic description of each refer to chapter-2)

- **A cough:** (productive or non-productive) usually worsen at night or early morning
- **Shortness of breath (SOB):** more noticeable when patient pause to breath while speaking.
- **Dyspnea:** described as chest tightness, more pronounced when lying down.
- **Cyanosis:** blue-gray or purplish discoloration of the mucous membranes
- **Anxiety and Panic**
- **Hyperventilation**
- **Tired and breathless**
- **Wheezing breath sound during expiration**
- **Use of accessory muscles during expiration and inspiration**
- **Pursed-lip breathing**
- **Increase Anteroposterior Chest Diameter or Barrel Chest**
- **Leaning forward**
- **Nasal flaring**

Cardiac symptoms of asthma:

Hypoxic stimulation of the carotid bodies of the peripheral chemoreceptors as the result of asthmatic episode sends the reflex signals to the respiratory muscles causes increase respiratory rate thereby enhances the speed of lung inflation that activates pulmonary reflex. Consequently, pulmonary reflex triggers tachycardia, cardiac output and blood pressure. The reason for increased cardiac output is to compensate for the hypoxemia resulted by shunting effects of the respiratory disorder. (For further detail explanation refer to chapter 2)

Etiologic Factors of Asthma

Asthma is divided into two classes according to the triggering factors:

- *Extrinsic asthma* is asthma caused by external or environmental agents.
- *Intrinsic asthma* occurs in the absence of or lack of evidence of an antigen –antibody reaction.

Extrinsic Asthma (Allergic or Atopic Asthma)

The asthmatic episode is clearly associated with exposure to a specific antigenic agent such as pollen, house dust, or feathers.

People with extrinsic asthma are said to have an allergic or atopic disorder, which means some hypersensitivity to common environmental allergens. Such individuals typically develop a wheal and flare reaction to a variety of skin allergens.

Extrinsic asthma is family related and usually appears in children and adults under the age of 30 years. This type of asthma often disappears after puberty.

Because extrinsic asthma is associated with an antigen-antibody-induced bronchospasm, an immunologic mechanism plays a major role in its induction. Like other organs, the lungs are protected against infection by certain immunologic mechanisms. Under normal circumstances, these mechanisms function without any clinical indication of their action. In people prone to extrinsic or allergic asthma, it is the immune response itself that creates the disease.

The Immunologic Mechanism

- Once a vulnerable person is exposed to a particular antigen, tissue cells of lymphoid develop specific IgE (reaginic) antibodies where they attach themselves to the surface of mast cells in the bronchial walls (Fig 4-3).

- Sustained exposure to the same antigen forms an antigen-antibody response on the surface of the mast cell, in turn, causes the mast cell degranulation and release chemical mediators such as histamine, a slow-reacting element of anaphylaxis (SRS-A), eosinophil chemotactic factor of anaphylaxis (ECF-A), and bradykinin (Fig 4-3).

- The release of these chemical mediators decreases the intracellular levels of cyclic adenosine monophosphate (cAMP) in the smooth muscles of the bronchi and results in bronchoconstriction. Moreover, these chemical mediators alter the permeability of capillaries, which results in the dilation of blood vessels and tissue edema (Fig 4-3).

- This antigen-antibody reaction is thought to trigger an asthmatic episode in individuals having extrinsic asthma. Furthermore, the production of IgE antibodies may be 20 times greater than normal in some asthmatic patients. (The normal IgE antibody level in the serum is about 200 ng/mL).

- Individuals with extrinsic asthma may demonstrate either a type I or a type III allergic response. The type I response is an immediate allergic reaction that is evoked by the antigen-antibody reaction just described. In a type III reaction, the invading antigen chemically combines with another precipitating immunoglobulin usually of the IgE class and delays the allergic response for 6 to 8 hours following exposure.

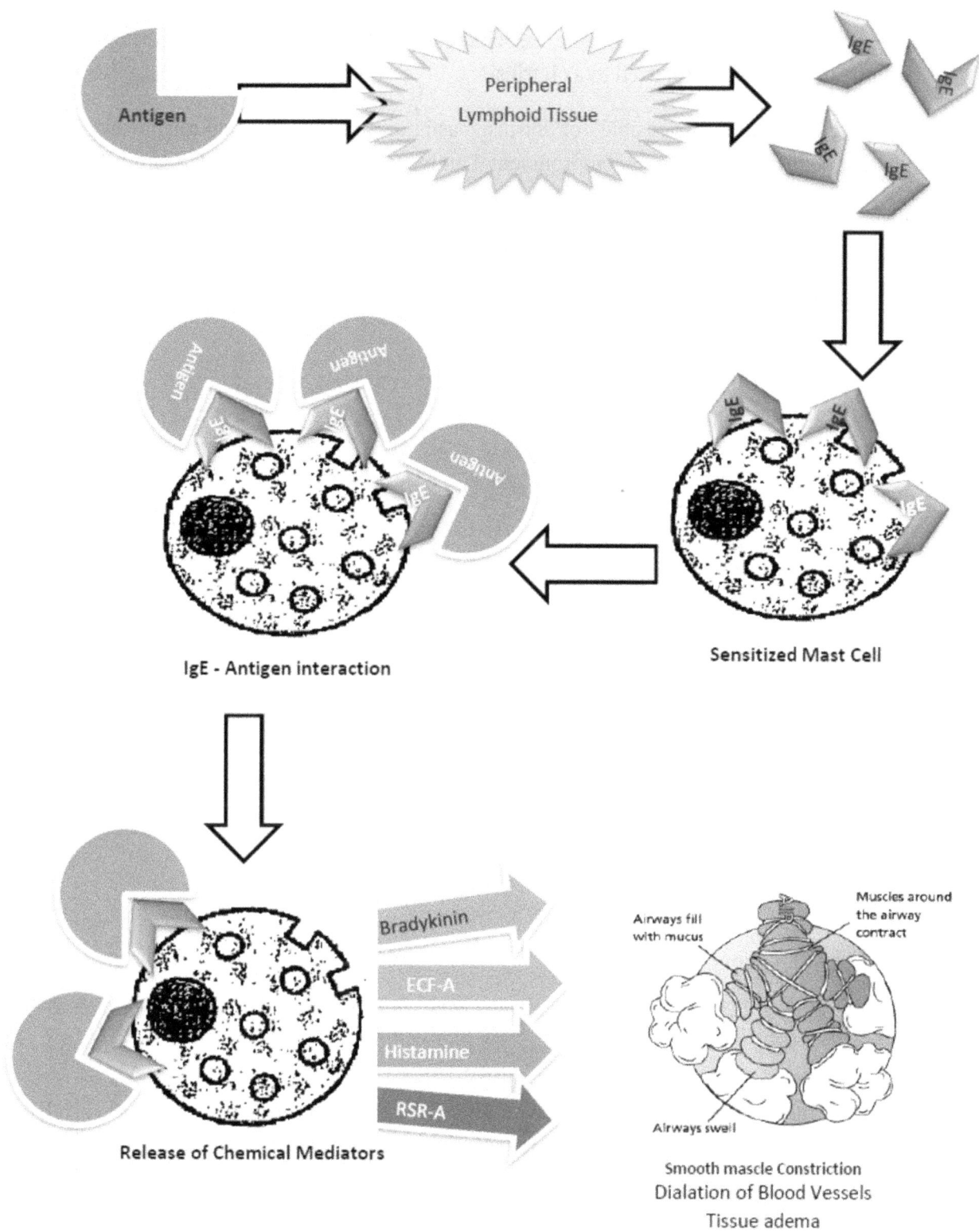

Figure 4-3 The immunologic mechanism of extrinsic asthma.

Intrinsic Asthma (Non-allergic or Non-Atopic Asthma)

When an asthmatic episode cannot be associated with the exposure to a specific external or environmental agent, it is referred to as intrinsic.

The etiologic features responsible for intrinsic asthma are elusive. Individuals with intrinsic asthma are not hypersensitive, to environmental antigens and have a normal serum IgE level.

Intrinsic asthma can be triggered by (1) infections, (2) cold air, (3) vapor, (4) industrial or occupational exposure, (5) chemical irritants or fumes, (6) dust and air pollutants, (7) tobacco smoke, (8) drugs (particularly aspirin), (9) emotional stress, and (10) exercise (Fig 4-4).

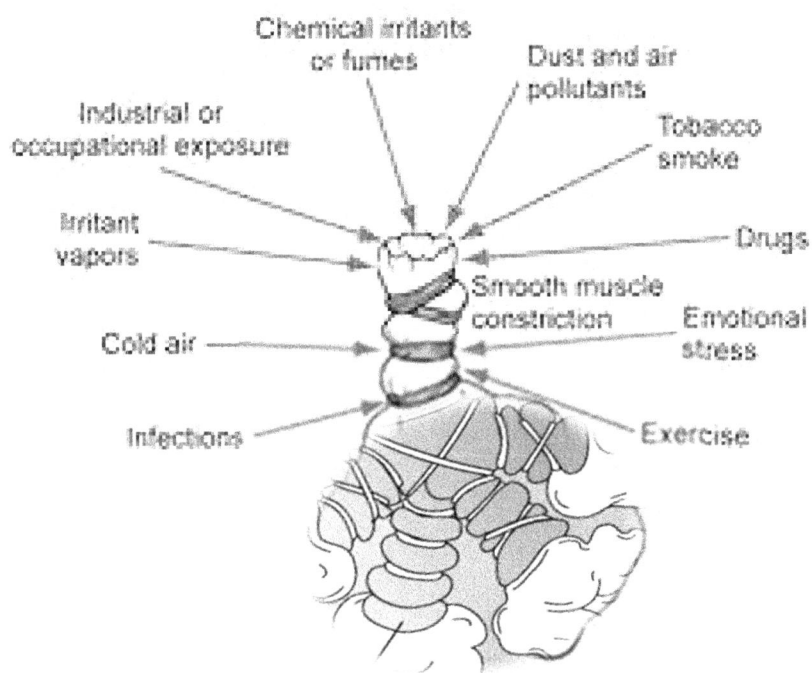

Figure 4-4: The etiologic factors of intrinsic asthma. Source: public domain images.search.yahoo.com,

The onset of intrinsic asthma usually occurs after the age of 35 years, and there is typically no family history of asthma. Chronic bronchitis is a frequent complication, as are bacterial and viral infections.

118

The β_2 – Blockade Theory of Intrinsic Asthma

It has been suggested that a partial β_2 – Blockade could account for the occurrence of asthma in some individuals. When the β_2 – receptors of the autonomic system are blocked, the cAMP level decreases, the cyclic guanosine monophosphate (cGMP) level increases and the bronchial smooth muscles constrict.

Chest Assessments and Diagnostic Findings

- **Chest Assessment Findings** (Chapter 2):
  - ➤ Diminished breath sounds due to air trapping
  - ➤ Wheezing, Crackles or Rhonchi due to narrowed airways, inflammation of the lining of the airways and excess mucus.
  - ➤ Percussion note displays hyper-resonant due to trapped air in the alveoli.
  - ➤ Decreased tactile and vocal fremitus caused by trapped air in the lungs.

- **Pulmonary Function Studies (PFT),** (diagnostic procedures chapter 2)

Table 4-1 The result of pulmonary function studies associated with asthma

Spirometry and Expiratory maneuver	Lung Volume and Lung capacity
↓ FVC	↑ VT
↓ $FEF_{200-1200}$	↑ RV
↓ $FEF_{25\%-75\%}$	↑ RV/TLC ratio
↓ FEV_T	↑ FRC
↓ FEV_1/FVC ratio	↑ CV
↓ MVV	↓ VC
↓ PEFR	↓ IRV
↓ $V_{max\ 50}$	↓ ERV

- **Arterial Blood Gas Analysis:** (Diagnostic procedures Chapter 2)

Table 4-2   The result of Arterial blood gas analysis associated with asthma

Initial Stages of an Asthmatic Episode	Progressive Stages of an Asthmatic Episode
Acute Alveolar Hyperventilation with Hypoxemia	**Acute Ventilatory Failure with Hypoxemia**
↓ PaO_2	↓ $PaO2$
↓ $PaCO_2$	↑ $PaCO2$
↓ HCO_3	↑ $HCO3$
↑ pH	↓ pH

- **Chest X-Ray Results Displays:**
  - ➢ Translucencies
  - ➢ Depressed or flattened diaphragm

During an asthma attack, residual volume, and functional residual capacity increases leading to alveolar hyperventilation that decreases the density of the lungs. Therefore, the x-ray appears darker than usual or translucent. Also, the increase in residual volume and functional residual capacity flattens and depresses the diaphragm. (As shown in fig. 4-5).

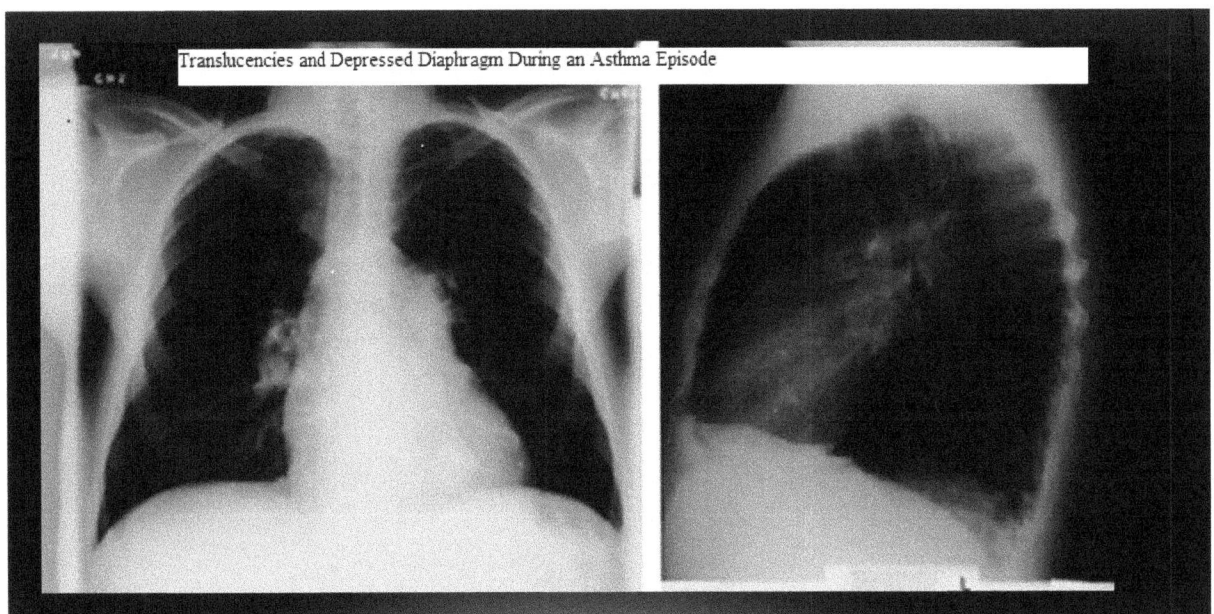

Figure 4-5 Chest X-Ray film of the lungs during an asthma episode. Source: Google images labeled for reuse.

Classification of asthma severity

Asthma severity is classified as severe persistent, moderate persistent, mild persistent and mild intermittent. These steps are essential in determining the appropriate treatment and initiation of the right therapy. (Table 4-3)

Table 4-3 Presenting Clinical features before treatment

Steps	Days with symptoms	Nights with symptoms	PEFR/FEV$_1$	PEF Variability
Step 4 Severe persistent	Continual	Frequent	≤ 60%	> 30%
Step 3 Moderate Persistent	Daily	≥ 5/month	> 60% - <80%	>30%
Step 2 Mild Persistent	3-6/week	3-4/month	≥ 80%	20-30%
Step 1 Mild intermittent	≤2/week	≤2/month	≥ 80%	< 20%

Treatment of Asthma

Control Environmental Triggers

Asthmatic patients should avoid the triggers commonly found at home, such as:
- ✓ Dust and dust mites found in draperies, bedding, linen, rugs, and furniture.
- ✓ Strong odor, spray and especially tobacco smoke.
- ✓ Feather pillows
- ✓ Mold and damp areas especially the basement
- ✓ Uncomfortable temperature and humidity

Anti-Asthma Medications

Types of medicines available for treating asthma are divided into two broad categories of **Relievers** and **Controllers**.

1. **Relievers** are bronchodilator drugs that relieve the symptoms of asthma such as a cough, chest tightness, breathlessness, and wheezing. The relievers are classified as Sympathomimetic (adrenergic), Parasympathetic (anticholinergics) and Xanthine bronchodilators.

Sympathomimetic Mechanism of Action

➢ Direct β2 stimulation, stimulate adenyl cyclase that increase cAMP thereby results in bronchodilation.
➢ Inhibits mediators release from mast cells.
➢ Increases ciliary activity resulting in increased mucus clearance
Sympathomimetic drugs are classified into selective β2-agonists and non-selective β-agonists as shown in Table 4-4.

Table 4-4 Classification of Sympathomimetic drugs

Selective β2-agonists	Non-selective β-agonists
Short Acting β2-agonists • **Salbutamol** (albuterol, Ventolin) inhalation, orally and I.V. • **Terbutaline** via inhalation, orally and S.C. • **levalbuterol** (Xopenex)) • **pirbuterol** (Maxair) ➢ Rapid onset of action 15-30 min ➢ Duration of action 4-6 hr. ➢ For acute asthmatic episode Long Acting β2-agonists • **Salmeterol** (Serevent, inhalation) • **Formoterol** (Foradil, inhalation) ➢ Long-acting bronchodilator 12hrs ➢ Low onset of action ➢ Not used for acute episodes ➢ Used for prophylaxis as nocturnal asthma ➢ Combined with inhaled corticosteroids to control asthma • **Advantages of β2-agonists** ➢ Minimal CVS side effect ➢ Appropriate for asthmatic patients with hypertension or heart conditions • **Disadvantages of β2-agonists** ➢ Skeletal muscle tremors ➢ Nervousness ➢ Tachycardia	**Epinephrine (isoprenaline)** ➢ Potent Bronchodilator ➢ Rapid Action within 15 minutes ➢ Aerosol Nebulizer or S.C. delivery ➢ Duration of action 60-90 minutes ➢ Drug of choice for acute anaphylaxis • **Disadvantages** ➢ Not effective orally ➢ Hyperglycemia in diabetes ➢ CVS side effect: tachycardia, arrhythmia, hypertension and angina ➢ Skeletal muscle tremor

Parasympatholytic (anticholinergic) agents also called Muscarinic antagonists
This agent inhibits bronchoconstriction and mucus secretion. Medications are used for acute severe asthma combined with β2-agonists and steroids. A most popular example of a non-selective muscarinic antagonist is ipratropium bromide or Atrovent and tiotropium or Spiriva administered via aerosol inhalation.

- **ipratropium bromide (Atrovent)**
- **tiotropium (Spiriva)**
  - ➢ A short-acting bronchodilator
  - ➢ Less effective than β2-agonists
  - ➢ No anti-inflammatory action
  - ➢ Minimal systemic side effects

Methyl-xanthine or xanthine bronchodilators
Xanthine are used to enhance bronchial smooth muscle relaxation
- ➢ Theophylline is given orally and parenterally
- ➢ Aminophylline (combination of theophylline and ethylenediamine) given orally and parenterally.

Mechanism of action
- ➢ Phosphodiesterase inhibitors
- ➢ ↑cAMP results in bronchodilation
- ➢ Adenosine receptors antagonists (A1)
- ➢ Increase diaphragmatic contraction
- ➢ Improves ventilation
- ➢ Stabilizes mast cell membrane

2. **Controllers** as the term suggest these drugs target the inflammatory process of asthma.

   Anti-inflammatory Agents
   These agents reduce the inflammation in the airways thereby lessen the spasm of the airways and bronchial hyper-reactivity.
   - ➢ Glucocorticoids
   - ➢ Mast cell stabilizers
   - ➢ Leukotrienes antagonists

   Glucocorticoids
   Glucocorticoids are given as prophylactic medications to reduce the frequency of asthma episodes. These agents are effective in allergic, exercise, antigen and irritant-induced asthma. An example of steroids used prophylactically is shown in Table 4-5.

   - ○ **Glucocorticoids Mechanism of Action**
     - ➢ Inhibition of phospholipase A2 decrease synthesis of arachidonic acid and prostaglandin and leukotrienes
     - ➢ Decrease inflammatory cells in airways such as macrophages and eosinophils